CW00369494

First Aid

Made Simple

The Made Simple series
has been created
especially for self-education
but can equally well
be used as
an aid to group study.
However complex the subject,
the reader is taken
step by step,
clearly and methodically,
through the course. Each volume
has been prepared by experts,
taking account of
modern educational requirements,
to ensure the most
effective way of
acquiring knowledge.

In the same series

Accounting
Acting and Stagecraft
Additional Mathematics
Administration in Business
Advertising
Anthropology
Applied Economics
Applied Mathematics
Applied Mechanics
Art Appreciation
Art of Speaking
Art of Writing
Biology
Book-keeping
Britain and the European
    Community
British Constitution
Business and Administrative
    Organisation
Business Calculations
Business Economics
Business Law
Business Statistics and Accounting
Calculus
Chemistry
Childcare
Child Development
Commerce
Company Law
Company Practice
Computer Programming
Computers and Microprocessors
Cookery
Cost and Management Accounting
Data Processing
Economic History
Economic and Social Geography
Economics
Effective Communication
Electricity
Electronic Computers
Electronics
English
English Literature
Financial Management
French
Geology
German
Graphic Communication

Housing, Tenancy and Planning
    Law
Human Anatomy
Human Biology
Italian
Journalism
Latin
Law
Management
Marketing
Mathematics
Metalwork
Modelling and Beauty Care
Modern Biology
Modern Electronics
Modern European History
Modern Mathematics
Modern World Affairs
Money and Banking
Music
New Mathematics
Office Administration
Office Practice
Organic Chemistry
Personnel Management
Philosophy
Photography
Physical Geography
Physics
Practical Typewriting
Psychiatry
Psychology
Public Relations
Public Sector Economics
Rapid Reading
Religious Studies
Russian
Salesmanship
Secretarial Practice
Social Services
Sociology
Spanish
Statistics
Technology
Teeline Shorthand
Twentieth-Century British History
Typing
Woodwork

First Aid

Made Simple

A.S. Playfair
MRCS, LRCP, DObst, RCOG

Illustrations by
Larry Pulley

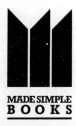

MADE SIMPLE
B O O K S

HEINEMANN : London

Copyright © 1986 A.S. Playfair

All rights reserved, including the right
of reproduction in whole or in part
in any form whatsoever

Printed and bound in Great Britain
by Richard Clay (The Chaucer Press) Ltd, Bungay, Suffolk
for the publishers, William Heinemann Ltd,
10 Upper Grosvenor Street, London W1X 9PA

This book is sold subject to the
condition that it shall not, by
way of trade or otherwise, be lent,
re-sold, hired out, or otherwise
circulated without the publisher's
prior consent in any form of binding
or cover other than that in which it is
published and without a similar condition
including this condition being imposed
on the subsequent purchaser

British Library Cataloguing in Publication Data

Playfair, A.S.
 First aid made simple.—(Made simple books,
 ISSN 0265-0541)
 1. First aid in illness and injury
 I. Title   II. Series
 616.02′52   RC87

ISBN 0-434-98604-6

Contents

Preface

The beginner may, perhaps, not realize that *First Aid* is exactly what the words state. It is help given immediately before full technical assistance arives.

First aid is surprisingly easy to learn. Another pleasant surprise is that, properly applied, its uncomplicated and logical steps can prove wonderfully effective, almost out of proportion to the work involved. The magic lies in knowing what to do, and in understanding the reason why. This book aims to teach those two things. No instructions will be given without explaining the principles involved.

On the other hand the book will not spend time and space on details of anatomy and physiology which, interesting as they may be, are not properly part of first aid.

Initially, we can consider just what is defined by the two words *First* and *Aid*.

First

Assistance is very definitely a preliminary one. The phrase 'First Aid' implies that it is to be followed by 'Second Aid', which is attended to by doctor or nurse. The first aider never usurps the role of these experts; his task is to put the patient in the best possible state until they take over. And this in turn involves a number of restrictions; the first aider realizes what he should not attempt. In fact he learns how effectively a minimum of acts can provide a maximum of protection.

Aid

Your help to patients has three main aims. *You must keep the patient alive.* Threat to life may be immediate as in the case of heavy bleeding or when breathing has stopped. There are also more hidden risks, like those run by the unconscious patient who is not properly positioned.

Not every case is as dramatically urgent as these. But it is true to say that the second aim applies to all injuries. *This is to prevent the condition from getting worse.* Dressing wounds and immobilizing fractures are good examples. Bad handling can considerably complicate the trouble.

Your third purpose is equally important: always *relieve pain, discomfort, and anxiety*. Treatment technique is designed to make the patient's physical suffering as slight as possible. But you will never forget that to a greater or lesser extent every injury creates psychological tension. The sympathetic and understanding manner with which you apply these techniques is of major importance. This is discussed in some detail in Chapters 9 and 22.

Equipment Needed

The last chapter advises on first aid kits. Equipment is important, but also it can delude you into a false sense of security. All too often you may find yourself called upon to help when no kit is available. You may waste valuable time trying to get one. Learn to improvize with the simple, everyday things which are at hand. You will find this stressed throughout the book.

Priorities in Learning

Subject order in this book is not an indication of relative importance and urgency. It is designed to make learning simpler and more successful.

Life saving techniques, such as artificial respiration, have the highest priority. However it is rare to have to use them. It is wise for the student to familiarize himself first with more common conditions before dealing with the relatively specialized matter of resuscitation, which is therefore given its logical learning order place in the middle of this book.

Unconsciousness is relatively common. However teaching the first aid involved comes more reasonably after a study of our breathing processes.

The index and the chapter headings will allow you to make rapid references in case of need. But you should read and learn the whole to reduce the necessity to look up. If your time is limited then at least make certain of having studied the following ten subjects (given here in alphabetical order).

Bleeding
Burns
Diabetes
Electric Shock
Epilepsy

Resuscitation
Road Accidents
Shock
Snakebites
Unconsciousness

With those understood you will already have become a very valuable person in an emergency. And then, when more time is available, you can complete your study of the remainder.

First Aid Classes

There are many organizations that run first aid classes, which are extremely interesting and well worth attending. These include a lot of practical exercises. The examination at the end of each course is fair and quite straightforward. Success establishes you as a qualified first aider. In Britain you can approach the St John's Ambulance Association (1 Grosvenor Crescent, London SW1) or the British Red Cross Society (9 Grosvenor Crescent, London SW1) and in Scotland the St Andrew's Ambulance Association (Milton Street, Glasgow C4). Their local addresses throughout the country can be found in the telephone book. Similar organizations exist all over the world.

Illustrations

The author is grateful to Larry Pulley for the combination of style and accuracy which features in his drawings.

1
Wounds

A wound implies damage to the skin, exposing underlying tissues. It seems a simple matter to protect it by covering. And so it is in the majority of cases. But a little thought shows that more may be involved, sometimes not very obviously. Approach any wound by considering the following possibilities.

Possible Complications

Is there heavy bleeding? You must control this immediately (see p. 27).

Could deeper structures be damaged? What shows as a small surface breach may overlie serious injury to an organ like the muscles, liver, lungs, bowels, and brain. Also a wound received through a hard blow could have caused a fracture. Sometimes a pierced blood vessel bleeds inside a limb, chest or abdomen: the blood may not show on the surface.

Is the patient at risk of developing shock? This important matter is dealt with on p. 100.

Infection is the threat to every wound. The way you do the dressing aims to reduce this risk to the minimum. Note that you do not use antiseptic lotions or creams on the wound. This would be the sphere of 'second', or medical, aid. Some antiseptics improperly used can irritate and can even hinder healing. They could also hinder any possible bacteriological tests that a doctor might wish to carry out.

Exceptionally your first aid may have to move into the 'second aid' field. You, and your badly wounded patient, could be in a remote area, days away from professional help. You will then use an antiseptic and very carefully follow exactly the instructions that accompany it. Any strong antiseptic will certainly kill microbes but could easily cause pain, damage to open tissues and to the body's defense mechanism against infection. Some liquid antiseptics are fine when prepared from freshly opened bottles, but once diluted to working strength will, after a time, gradually become not only ineffective but also contaminated.

A wise expedition leader will have got a doctor's advice about the antiseptic to include in his kit.

General Wound Treatment

In this chapter it will be assumed that bleeding is slight. It will be controlled by a dressing firmly and correctly applied.

Treatment may be modified according to circumstances but the general principles are:

1. Loosely cover the wound area temporarily with clean light material, such as a piece of surgical gauze or the inside surface of a clean handkerchief (see p. 12).

2. Lie or sit the patient down. But be careful if he has received a severe blow, which could have caused a fracture; do not move him until you have safeguarded the possible fracture (see pp. 68–71).

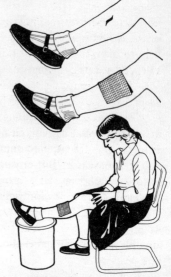

3. Wash your hands.

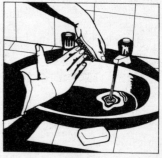

4. Collect all the equipment you need. Place it on a clean towel or handkerchief.

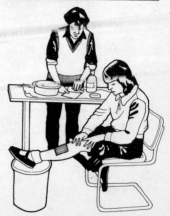

5. Remove any *loose* foreign matter (glass, metal, gravel) from the surface by lightly brushing with a clean cloth or swab of gauze. But do not try to remove anything *embedded* in the wound (see p. 4). Also do not disturb any blood clot for this could start the bleeding again.

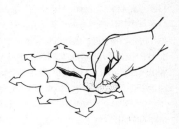

6. Gently clean *the skin around* the wound with soap and water. Do this with dampened (not dripping) swabs of wool or gauze or with clean cloth. Do not clean the open wound itself, and try to avoid getting any liquid on to the wound, using a fresh swab or a fresh part of the cloth for each stroke.

7. Touching the material only by its edges, cut gauze to a size large enough not only to cover the wound but also to extend well over the surrounding skin. Hold it by the corners and lower it over the wound.

8. Cover this with a *thick* pad of gauze or suitable material. Now bandage the whole gently, but firmly enough to make sure that the dressing will not slip later. Secure the bandage with a knot, or use adhesive tape, or safety pin. To avoid unpleasant pressure on the wound make sure these are not over the wound site itself. The Prepared Sterile Dressing (see p. 14), combining gauze, pad and bandage, is the ideal to use if it is available. See also pp. 11–15 concerning types of dressings.

Bandage
Pad
Dressing

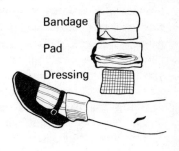

9. If the wound is an extensive one on a limb, rest the part in a slightly raised position. This is comfortable and reduces swelling. You can put an arm in a sling. But do not move any part you suspect to be fractured until

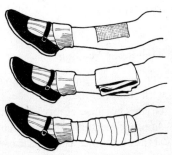

you have protected the fracture (see p. 70).

10. If necessary take anti-shock measures (see p. 105).

Object Embedded in Wounds

Do not try to remove anything firmly embedded in a wound, for its movement may do more damage. Lay a dressing (e.g. gauze) loosely over the wound and the object. Then over this place a ring pad (see p. 17) so that the object lies within its centre. The ring pad forms a protecting frame over which you can put the main dressing pad and then bandage the pad down without pressing on the object itself.

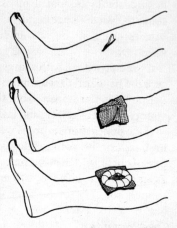

Alternatively you can improvize a built-up dressing to form a raised framework round the wound.

Sometimes instead of the ring pad you can improvize with a protective cup over the gauze and under the bandage. It can vary in size and nature from a small pill box to a plastic yoghurt or cream container— well cleaned, of course. The complete dressing may look misshapenly lumpy, but that does not matter.

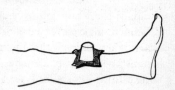

If the protruding object is too big to be covered, pack dressings closely all round it and apply the bandage so that it comes close to but not over the object.

Abdominal Wounds

The main danger is damage to organs with internal bleeding (see p. 36). Urgent hospital admission is needed. Another danger is protrusion of some of the abdominal contents through the wound; the risk is lessened if the abdominal walls are relaxed, for this allows the wound to remain more closed.

To obtain this relaxation put the patient on his back, half propped up, with head and shoulders elevated on large cushions or folded blankets or coats. Keep his knees and hips well bent by similar objects under the knees.

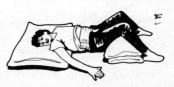

Cover the wound with a large clean material pad and bandage. Make sure the bandage does not press tightly on it through the dressing.

If anything protrudes from the wound do *not* interfere with it. Let your covering be moist, and take care that the bandage is not too tight.

If the patient vomits or loses consciousness you will have to turn him on his side with his head low, to avoid the danger of fluid or vomit passing back into the windpipe. The position is similar to the Recovery Position (see p. 112) but with both knees bent.

Chest Wounds

See p. 51.

Eye Wounds

(Chemicals in the eye: see p. 98)
Warn the patient that pain may increase if the eyeball moves. Make him lie down. In this case you must *not* try to wash round the wound for this could further damage the eyeball. Cover the eye (closed if possible) with a soft pad extending to the forehead and cheek. Bandage lightly over this. If anything projects from the eyeball, which might get pressed on by the bandage, treat it as you would a wound with an embedded object (see p. 4). If the patient is restless it may be wise to cover the good eye as well since its movement entails the movement of the injured eye; explain to the patient

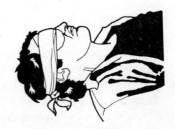

why you are doing this.

Send him to hospital as soon as possible.

Animal and Insect Bites

See pp. 165–70.

Bullet and Shrapnel Wounds

Bullets can do a great deal of damage to deeper structures, and internal bleeding (p. 36) could be one of the more severe complications.

A missile may only make a small wound as it hits the skin. But, deflected by the resistance of the tissues, it tends to track a widening path through the body. If it comes out it will do so through a relatively large hole.

In the case of such injuries always look gently and carefully for the possible exit wound as well as the entrance wound. Both must be dressed. If you find the missile which has come out, retrieve it; wrap it carefully in clean material or paper and hand it to the authorities who take charge. Handle it as little as possible.

Bruises

Bruises are not proper wounds since they happen under intact skin. A blow to some part of the body, a sudden stretch (as in a severe sprain) or any disruption of tissue can easily break blood vessels. Even if these vessels are small, blood escapes and collects under the skin, to give a purple discolouration soon after the injury. Over the next few days the stagnant blood undergoes some chemical action which produces greenish or yellow tinges.

Bruising does not always appear directly over the injured site. It could show a little lower, for the blood may ooze downwards a short distance under the skin. For instance, a broken bone at the ankle could be followed by bruising on the foot.

There is no true first aid treatment for the fully formed bruise. But immediately after the injury you might reduce bruising by cooling the area concerned so as to contract the blood vessels.

Cool by applying a cold compress (see p. 62) to the injured part. At the same time keep it rested and raised if possible. But do this fairly quickly, certainly within the first thirty or forty minutes after the injury. After that time the bleeding is likely to have filled up adjacent tissues and then stopped.

A cold compress given later could relieve pain, but is unlikely to affect the extent of the bruise.

The Pattern Bruise is the name given to bruise marks left by items through which a blow's impact was received. Braces, the weave of clothes, belt, buckles, buttons or brassière fastenings are all examples: objects in pockets and jewellery on the skin are others. The marks may appear slight and immediate discomfort be minimal, so that the patient tends to ignore them.

However, you must not disregard them. Any blow strong enough to create these skin patterns may have been strong enough to have damaged an internal organ. Your patient may perhaps be bleeding internally. Make him rest and get medical advice at once.

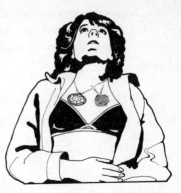

Bruise from blow through pendant.

Crush Injuries

If part of the body is caught and held down by the fall of a heavy object there are risks of fractures and of wounds with heavy bleeding. There will be, as well, less obvious, but considerable, damage to deep tissues. The rupture of many small blood vessels can produce extensive bruising, i.e. blood taking up space under the skin. Also there will be a great deal of oozing out of the thin clear fluid part of the blood (plasma) from unbroken vessels in the area.

The total effect can be that of swelling and hard pressure which impedes circulation. For instance if a thigh is pinned down by a heavy weight the life of the rest of the leg beyond it may be at risk from the reduced blood supply.

When the limb is released it may at first appear normal in size. But soon after it could swell up as the fluids now fill up the tissues. There are two other likely consequences. The immediate one is that the loss of so much fluid and blood is likely to bring the patient into a state of shock. A more delayed

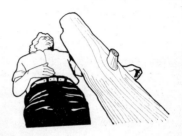

danger comes from a number of harmful chemicals which are produced in the damaged area. After release these can pass into the circulation and eventually damage the patient's kidneys.

First Aid for Minor Cases

There may be, for example, a hand or foot which was quickly released.

1. Control any severe bleeding (p. 27).
2. Protect any likely fracture (p. 70).
3. Keep the part elevated.
4. Apply a cold compress (p. 62).

These last two measures help to reduce the degree of swelling.

5. Get medical help.

First Aid for Major Cases

There may be, for example a leg or an arm where crushing under a very heavy weight has lasted half an hour or more.

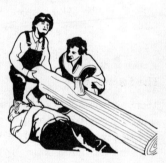

1. At once control any severe bleeding (p. 27).

2. Get the heavy weight removed as soon as possible.

3. Keep the patient lying down with his head low. If it is safe to move the legs at this stage get them raised on some support like cushions or rolled up blankets or over a low stool or box. This helps to counter shock.

4. Rapidly protect any possible fracture by immobilizing the damaged limb (p. 71). Of course you should do this first to a leg before elevating. You may have to improvize splint and padding quite quickly.

5. Get an injured limb raised on a suitable support. This helps to reduce the swelling.

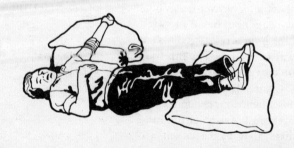

6. Cover any open wounds with only quite a light dressing. The less covering there is to a crush injury the better: by warming up that area thick covering would dilate the blood vessels and increase the oozing from them.

7. Cover the rest of the patient to guard against heat loss (p. 105).

8. Watch him closely lest he lose consciousness. In this case you must try to place him in as near the Recovery Position (p. 112) as his injuries allow.

9. Get him to hospital by stretcher as soon as possible. Send with him a written message telling at what time he was crushed and at what time he was released.

10. If there is any delay in getting him to hospital and if he is conscious give him sips of cold or tepid (not hot) water.

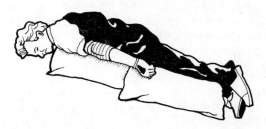

The Tetanus Risk

Many wounds carry the risk of tetanus ('lockjaw') infection. The causative microbes can survive a long time as spores are resistant to the heat or drying that would kill ordinary germs. Inside wounds, offering them new conditions of humidity, nutrition and temperature, the spores may resume their dangerously active forms, especially in wounds with much contamination and tissue damage.

The microbes and spores, often present in animal dung and in soil, are particularly common in agricultural regions. But ordinary road dust and private gardens can harbour them; also infection might arise from animal bites or even the prick of a rose thorn. Those at risk range from the child at play to the explorer, from the person peeling potatoes to the mechanic repairing a car.

Tetanus produces a poison which attacks nerves and brain, causing painful muscle spasm and interfering with breathing and heart action. Symptoms may appear within a few days after the accident; rarely the illness takes much longer to develop.

Everyone, from babyhood onwards should be immunized, by a course of simple, harmless injections. The protection given lasts for five to ten years after which a single repeat injection can extend the protection.

Even so any injury, from animals or contaminated by soil or dust, is a matter for medical advice. Deep puncture wounds are particularly dangerous since the microbe thrives in the absence of air. Whenever the circumstances warrant, always urge your patient to consult his doctor.

Amputations

First you will deal with the open stump, covering it with a dressing and controlling bleeding by pressure.

Next retrieve the severed part if you can and send it to hospital with the patient; not only finger tips but even large parts can sometimes be replanted. The severed part must not dry, it should be kept cold and it must be protected. Put it in a clean, well-closed, plastic bag. If possible place this within a second plastic bag, containing ice. Put the whole in a labelled, firm container and hand to the ambulance attendant. Try to notify the hospital in advance that this has been done, so that appropriate measures can be prepared.

Questions

1. A man is found held down by a heavy metal door which fell on his leg about forty minutes ago. How should he be helped?

2. At a picnic a young woman stumbles against a wire fence. A piece of the metal breaks off and gets deeply stuck in her ankle projecting about ½ centimetre above the skin.

Describe in detail the first aid and advice you give.

3. You see a pedestrian hit by a car which backed hard into him. He appears fit and active but very angry because this smashed a watch in his waistcoat pocket, bruising his skin. He says he is going to the police station to complain. What do you do?

4. Explain your opinion about the place of antiseptics in the first aid treatment of wounds.

2
Dressings and Bandages

This chapter is mainly for reference and for reminder. A student on his own should read through this at least once to get a general view of many ways in which dressings exist and can be used. Experience and practice soundly reinforce this, especially in first-aid classes.

Obtainable from chemists' shops, dressings, neatly packed and ready for use, are invaluable ... if they are to hand at the time of the accident. The most important lesson is that of *improvization*. There is practically no dressing equipment that cannot be improvized from simple domestic material. At each stage some examples are given; you will be able to think of others. And when an emergency arises far away from any first-aid kit you will discover how quickly inventive you can be.

As described in Chapter 1 an ideal dressing for a wound consists of three things: a clean cover, a pad overlying it and a bandage securing the whole.

The Clean Cover

This should, if possible, come from a freshly opened pack. Cut and position it with the least possible handling keeping your fingers (and anything else) off the surface which is going on the wound.

White gauze is the usual dressing and is available in quite small packs. The *perforated film absorbent* (P.F.A.) dressings available in sizes 5 sq. cm, 10 sq. cm and 10 cm × 20 cm are very handy. They are sterile and packed individually in protective envelopes. By opening and handling

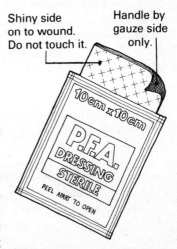

Shiny side on to wound. Do not touch it.

Handle by gauze side only.

10 cm x 10 cm

P.F.A. DRESSING STERILE

PEEL APART TO OPEN

carefully the envelope and the back of the dressings you can place them on, without touching the surface of the dressing which goes on the wound. This surface is a shiny one: it looks waterproof but in fact is absorbent. It is the plain surface that you can hold.

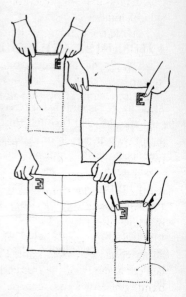

You can improvize dressings from clean handkerchiefs, small towels or pillowcases. Hold the article at two corners by the tips of thumb and index finger and let it fall open. Still holding only at corners refold it to the correct size so that what was the inside surface now becomes the outer one. Untouched by hand this fresh surface goes on the wound. A pillow case is useful for encasing a whole limb.

Do not use cotton wool or fluffy material like lint directly on a wound; it is too rough and shreddy, with a tendency to stick.

The Pad

Cotton wool is customary; it should, if possible, be from a freshly opened pack.

Gamgee tissue consists of a thickness of cotton wool sandwiched between outer layers of gauze; these layers restrict the thready shredding of the wool. *Improvizing pads is easily done by folding thickly together any suitable clean soft material, such as handkerchiefs, towels, socks.*

The Bandage

Plain white roller bandages are the usual ones. But *conforming bandages* and *elastic bandages* have more 'give' and are easier to adapt round uneven contours. They also help more to give firm pressure. But their elastic pressure can easily become excessive. Take great care not to put them on so tightly that they interfere with the circulation.

Most plain bandages come in regulation widths: 2.5 cm (for fingers); 5 cm and 7.5 cm (for head and limbs); 10 cm and 15 cm (for abdomen or chest).

The rules of good bandaging are simple:

1. Get the patient comfortable with the injured part firmly supported.

2. Stand in front rather than to one side of him.

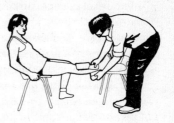

3. Hold the bandage so that its roll is uppermost in your hand.

4. Apply the bandage from below upwards.

5. Start with a firm (but not tight) turn.

6. Then let each successive turn cover two-thirds of the preceding turn.

7. Carry the bandage, to at least its width, above the top of the dressing. For neatness fold the end of the bandage under itself.

8. Fasten it with a safety pin, with adhesive tape or by a knot. For this last cut a length of the free end of the bandage down its centre. Knot together at their base the two 'tapes' thus created, and tie them round the limb.

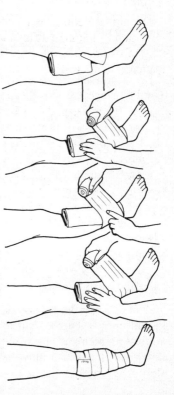

On a limb it is important not to make the bandage so tight that it will compress blood vessels and interfere with circulation. Unless the nature of the wound prevents this, leave toes and finger tips free and visible so that you can note any dusky discolouration from an impeded blood supply. If you do see this undo the bandage and reapply it less tightly.

Warn the patient to report if his hand or foot becomes white, dusky, swollen or numb; these signs might indicate a need to reapply the bandage.

There are many things from which you can improvize bandages: socks, stockings, towels, thin belts, scarves and neckties are examples.

Adhesive strapping can be used to hold gauze and padding on the skin if no suitable bandaging is available.

Prepared sterile dressings are extremely convenient, ready for use, combinations of gauze, pad, and bandage. Layers of gauze backed by cotton wool are attached near the end of the roller bandage. After you have broken the protective wrapping be careful not to touch the gauze: you handle only the bandage.

These dressings come in three sizes. In practice the medium and the large sizes are the useful ones.

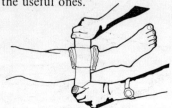

Adhesive dressings are very suitable for small superficial wounds and come either as continuous strips to be cut to size or as single dressings of different sizes.

They consist of an adhesive backing which extends beyond the edges of the gauze pad attached to it. In front are two protective strips which you *partly* peel off to expose the gauze.

Without touching the gauze put the dressing over the wound. Now carefully complete peeling off the strips and press down the edges of the dressing. The skin must be dry for the dressing to hold.

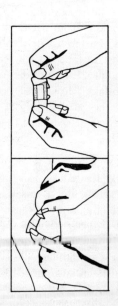

Tubular Gauze Bandage

Instead of being flat this bandaging comes as a long tube from which an appropriate length is cut for each dressing. It is made in various widths to match any part of the body from little toe to chest. For first aid you need consider only the smallest sizes suitable for fingers and toes.

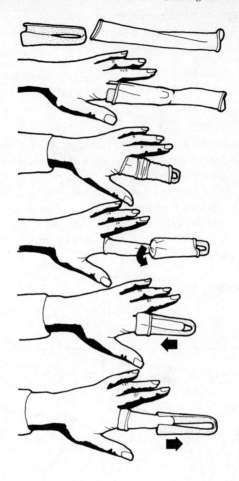

1. Cut off a length of bandage slightly longer than twice the length to be covered.

2. Fit an open end of the bandage over the top of the special two-pronged metal or plastic applicator. Push it down to the applicator's base.

3. Slip the applicator with its bandage over the whole of the finger.

4. Now withdraw the applicator, while holding the bandage in position on the finger.

5. When you have got the applicator just clear of the finger tip give it a couple of turns, twisting the tubular bandage at this point.

6. Push the applicator back over the finger. It will carry with it a

second layer of bandaging.

7. You can secure the base of the bandage to the finger with adhesive tape.

If you wish to leave the top of the finger visible: at stage 4 withdraw the applicator to only just below the finger tip, and leave out stage 5.

Making Knots

In all first-aid work you should always use the *reef knot*, which is firm and flat and does not slip. Also it is more comfortable for the patient. Try to avoid having it press against a bony part or over an injured area. When necessary you can put soft padding underneath it. Pick up end A, pass it over and then tuck it round and under end B. Pull it firm. This is half the knot. Now again pick up end A, pass it over and then tuck it round and under end B. This completes the knot, which you now pull tight.

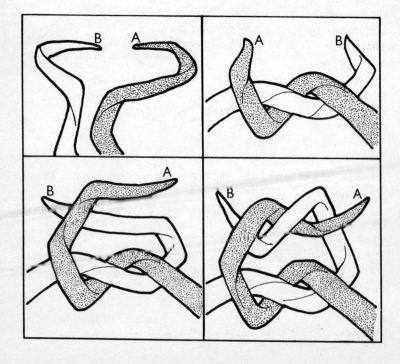

Tuck the ends tidily out of sight.

The whole can be summed up by the phrase 'right over left; then left over right'. (But if you find it easier you can do it the other way round, interchanging right and left.)

Triangular Bandages

These, a mainstay of first-aid kits for many decades, are immensely useful for their versatility. They take little space and do many things. Most are made from calico or linen; some, for 'once-only' use, are of toughened paper. Also they can be obtained sterile in individual packs and, therefore, are suitable, if carefully handled, to place directly on a wound.

You can make triangular bandages by cutting diagonal pieces of material not less than one metre (or one yard) square. Also you can improvize by folding a towel or large scarf suitably.

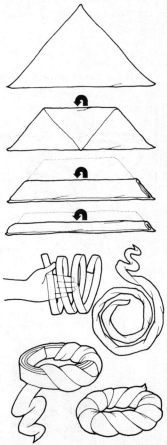

They can be used in the form of a sling (see p. 18) or opened fully for keeping a large dressing in position. They can be folded to make broad or narrow bandages.

For the *broad bandage* fold the point to meet the centre of the base and then fold the bandage again in the same direction.

For the *narrow bandage* fold once again in the same direction.

For the *ring pad* (see p. 17) pass one end of a narrow bandage once or twice round your fingers, then bring the other end of the bandage through the loop you have made. Continue to pass it through and through until the whole of the bandage is used and a firm ring made. Tuck in the end.

You can also make ring pads of different sizes from handkerchiefs, or from small towels and scarves which have been folded into narrow form.

The Sling

The sling is a band of material passed round the neck and looped over the chest to support an injured arm. (It is also used in some cases of chest injury.) Triangular bandages lend themselves admirably to this.

It is important that you slip the sling into position without disturbing the arm. Make sure that, until the sling is secured and takes the weight, the injured part is well steadied. The patient may be able to do this. Ideally he should be sitting or lying. (For clarity this support is not shown in the following illustrations.)

The Arm Sling

1. Ensure that the patient's hand is a little higher than the elbow.
2. Bring the upper end of the sling well over the shoulder of the injured side.
3. Get the point of the sling clear of the elbow.
4. Make sure that the patient's fingers are free and visible so that their colour can be checked to confirm that there is no obstruction to the circulation.
5. Bring up the lower end of the sling and knot it to the upper end to support the whole of the arm. Make sure that the knot is in the hollow above the collar bone.
6. Fold the point forward and pin it to the front of the sling.

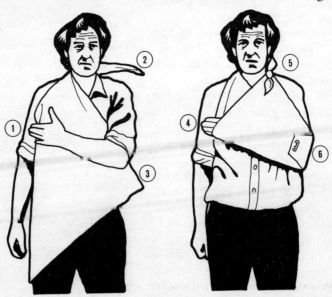

The Elevation Sling

Use this when a hand, chest or shoulder is badly injured or when firm support to the forearm is needed.

1. Have the hand on the chest with the fingers near the shoulder.
2. Place the bandage over the forearm with its point far beyond the elbow.
3. Tuck the base well under the hand, forearm, and elbow.
4. Bring the lower end under the bent elbow and round the patient's back to the opposite shoulder. You may have to adjust the height of the sling to fit.
5. Tie the ends together in the hollow above the collar bone.
6. Tuck the point between the forearm and the front of the bandage and fix it with a safety pin.

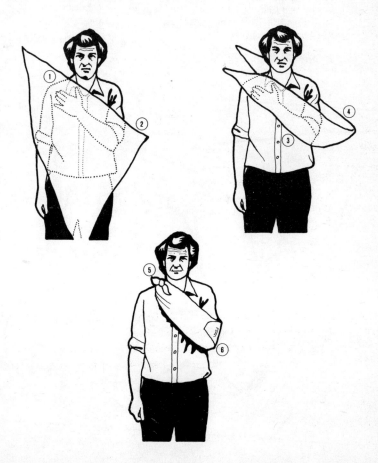

Improvized Slings

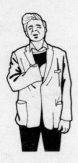 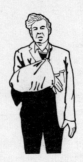 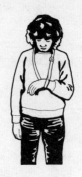

Hand inside buttoned up coat; sleeve pinned to lapel

Bottom edge of coat turned up and pinned to opposite lapel.

Belt, braces, necktie or tapes.

Using Triangular Bandages to Cover Various Sites

Scalp

Fold over a 'hem' at the base.

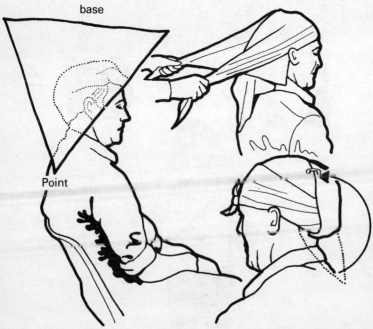

Hand

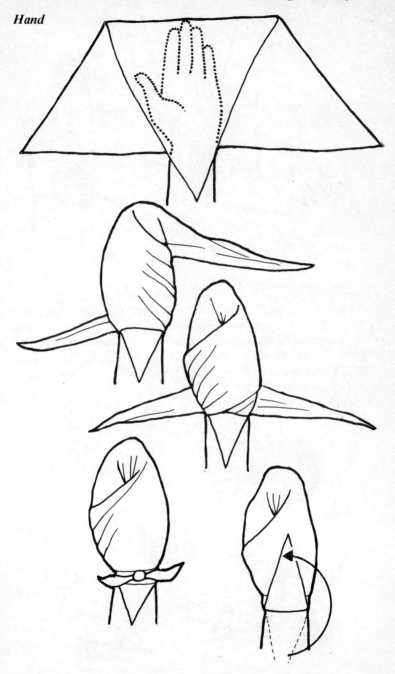

Foot

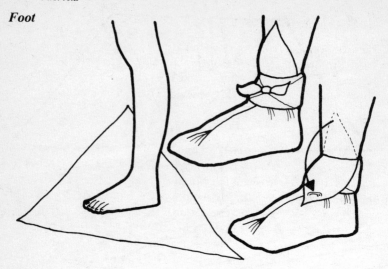

Figure of Eight Bandage

This bandage very usefully goes around the upper and lower aspects of a joint like the elbow or the ankle. A common use in first aid is that of tying ankles together as part of the immobilization of a fractured leg.

The two ankles lie side by side. Place the centre of the bandage behind both legs just above the ankles. Bring the ends forward over the feet and one of the ends under the soles. (If shoes are worn make the bandage lie against the projection of the heel.) Make sure that the bandage is firm (not tight) and tie the knot by the side of the foot of the uninjured leg.

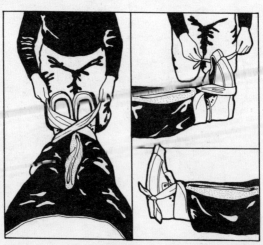

Bandaging Limbs

There always is a risk of bandaging arm, leg, finger or even toe not merely firmly but so tightly that this interferes with the blood flow or presses hard on a nerve. After a while the patient feels discomfort or pain. Yet he may not report this, believing it to be the consequence of his injury.

You can take care in two ways.

1. After any bandaging check the colour of the limb extremity, or tip of finger or toe. If it is pale or dusky blue the circulation is probably impeded. If the colour seems fair you can make a test. Press a toenail or fingernail hard with your finger. As soon as you release pressure the nail area will look pale. But if the circulation is normal, colour will return to it very fast, within two or three seconds. If it takes markedly longer suspect that your bandage is too tight.

2. Always warn the patient that, should the limb beyond the bandage become puffy, painful, numb, pale or discoloured, he must report it at once. If he is alone he can loosen the bandage a little, but then should get it seen to as soon as possible for readjusting.

Questions

1. Describe the different sorts of dressings and bandaging you could use for a wound of the thumb.

2. You are dressing a severely cut arm. What precautions do you take to avoid the patient suffering from tight bandaging.

3. Towards the end of a small wedding reception in a church hall a guest slips and falls heavily on his right arm. Also he has a deep cut of the hand and another in the forearm from a broken champagne glass, but fortunately they are not bleeding severely and nothing is embedded in the wounds. A set of bandages and dressings is not available. Describe in detail how you cope with the injuries.

4. What is the advantage of the elastic bandage? And what is its disadvantage? What are your precautions as you apply it?

5. The average dressing is described as having three components. What are they? In the absence of a first-aid kit how could you improvize these components?

3
Blood and Bleeding

Blood's main task is carrying oxygen to all tissues, for without oxygen they would die. Circulation of the blood is intimately linked with the action of the lungs.

About one-fifth of the air we breathe consists of oxygen. At each chest inspiration air reaches the many minute sacs which form the lungs. Here oxygen passes through the delicate lining of these sacs into the blood coursing through the microscopic vessels that serve them.

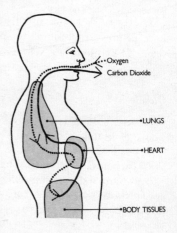

Enriched by oxygen the blood passes on to the heart which then pumps it round the body. The tissues extract oxygen; their life processes 'burn' it up and convert it to carbon dioxide. This is now taken away by the blood which returns to the heart, and is pumped back to the lungs.

Now the carbon dioxide passes into the air sacs, and is released out to the atmosphere as air is breathed out from the chest.

The Heart Pump

The blood passes through the hollow chambers which form the heart, chambers whose walls are powerful muscles. Heart beats are formed by the contraction and relaxation of the muscles, pumping blood through the vessels all round the body. In adults at rest this beat is normally at the rate of 60 to 80 times a minute, but exercise or emotion can send it higher, even up to about 120. Children have a faster rate at rest—up to 100 a minute. The new-born baby has a rate of about 120 to 140. In fevers and in some heart disorders the rate increases.

The Pulse

Each heart beat sends an impulse into arteries and some of these can be easily felt as the pulse. The pulse's rate and strength therefore give a good indication of how fast and well the patient's heart is beating.

The pulse is best tested where an artery lies close under the skin and also just over a bone against which it can be gently pressed by the examiner's finger. Three arteries lend themselves very well to this: at the wrist, by the ear and at the side of the neck. Choose the most suitable area for the circumstances, remembering to disturb the patient as little as possible.

Feel with fingers and not with thumb, which is less sensitive. Do not press your fingers more than is needed to be able to note:

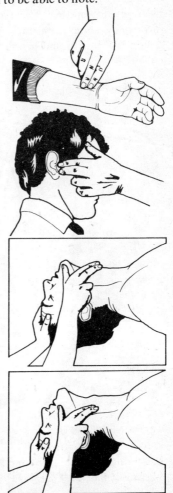

(a) the rate per minute (count for 15 seconds and multiply the result by 4);

(b) the regularity or evenness of beat;

(c) the strength.

At the Wrist

Put the tips of two or three fingers at the front of the wrist, a little above its crease and at the thumb side.

If you bend the patient's hand a little forward it relaxes tendons which pass across the wrist and makes it easier to feel the pulse.

At the Ear

Put one or two fingers immediately in front of the notch of the ear.

In the Neck

You will get the position correctly if first you put your fingers lightly on the patient's 'Adam's Apple', the hard projection of the larynx ('voice box') in the front of the neck. Then slide them sideways to where the artery lies in the hollow of the neck. Feel down gently.

There is little point in assessing a patient's pulse unless you are quite familiar with the normal sensation. Practice regularly on all ages and types of people.

The heart's behaviour, and therefore the pulse, may change as the patient's condition worsens or improves. In some circumstances you may have to take his pulse at regular intervals (say five to fifteen minutes) and record your findings against the time. This information may be useful to the doctor who takes over.

Blood Function and Volume

It would be a great mistake to think of blood only in terms of oxygen carriage. A very great number of substances travel in it from one part of the body to another. Chemical messengers (called hormones) are formed by some important glands to reach and influence distant structures. Nutritional products like glucose are taken to tissues as

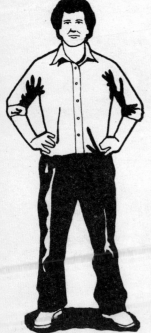
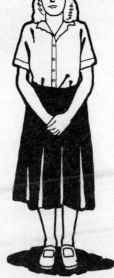
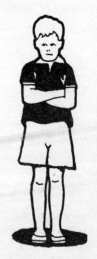

11 STONE WEIGHT
11 PINTS OF BLOOD

8 STONE WEIGHT
8 PINTS OF BLOOD

5 STONE WEIGHT
5 PINTS OF BLOOD

70 KG WEIGHT
6 LITRES OF BLOOD

50 KG WEIGHT
4½ LITRES OF BLOOD

30 KG WEIGHT
2½ LITRES OF BLOOD

essential for their function. Unwanted products are carried to organs like the liver and kidneys, which dispose of them. Millions of circulating blood cells regulate processes like the oxygen exchanges and the defence against infection.

Blood is to the body what the traffic on roadways is to the well-being of the state. Raw goods are brought to factories; food and manufactured goods are delivered to stores; shoppers take them to homes and larders; civil and armed services protect against disruption and attend to repairs.

If transport is interrupted or weakened the people of towns and villages would suffer. In the same way the body is at risk if there is depletion or blockage of the blood supply. The brain is particularly sensitive in this way, and this includes the nerve centres which control basic life functions such as heart beat, lung action and blood pressure, and temperature regulation.

The body automatically and rapidly compensates for small blood losses, but will be in danger when the bleeding is heavy. The illustrations show, very approximately, the likely total volume of blood in people of different weights.

In accidents with severe bleeding several litres or pints could be lost very fast unless effective first aid was given at once.

Stopping Bleeding

Blood escaping from broken blood vessels at wounds tends to clot. It changes from being a fluid and becomes jelly like, and then almost solid. Given the right circumstances this clot forms in a very few minutes, plugging the wound and the vessels and preventing further bleeding.

This happens spontaneously if bleeding is slight and slow. But where a large vessel is involved the flow is fast and powerful. The clot material is constantly washed away before it forms and has a chance to get fixed. The first-aider's task is to press on the wound and block the bleeding, or at least to slow it down considerably. He maintains pressure until good clotting has taken place. At the same time he takes care to protect his patient with anti-shock measures (see p. 105).

Mild Bleeding

This will be controlled if you treat it as a wound, with a well-applied dressing (see p. 11).

Severe, Dangerous Bleeding

All too often the victim watches with helpless horror as his blood escapes. You have to take charge at once. Do not spend time washing your hands; in this case speed is much more important than cleanliness.

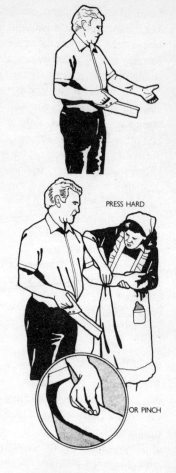

Immediately press on the wound. You can use finger and thumb to pinch the wound edges very firmly together. Or, if this is more suitable, press your palm and fingers down on the wound. You must not let go: maintain this pressure all the time during the next steps.

Do not ask the patient to apply the pressure himself while you go to seek dressings and help. He could become very anxious if left alone. Understandably he may also be in too poor a state to press correctly and strongly.

Still holding on to the wound get the patient sitting or (better) lying down. Reassure him by telling him you are getting the trouble under control. If you are dealing with a limb try to keep it raised for this can decrease its blood flow a little. But you may have to avoid this movement if you suspect that it is fractured.

You have now to replace:

1. *your hand* with a thick pad and;
2. *the pressure* of your hand with a firm bandage.

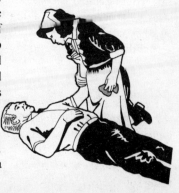

Look about for improvized material.
With your free hand get hold of what
you could use: handkerchief, scarf,
towel, napkin, necktie, stocking and
so on.

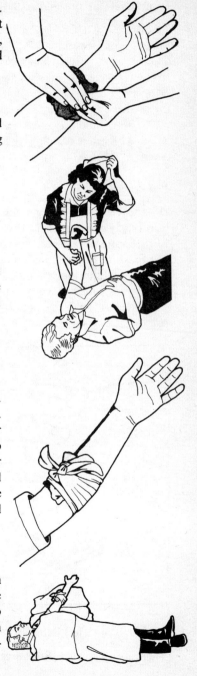

Slip a thick and bunched-up pad
under your hand which is still pressing
down.

Take and shape your improvized
bandage. Carefully wind it over the
pad, keeping this pressed down, and
make the knot directly over the pad.

Bleeding should now be controlled.
But you cannot be entirely sure.
Watch your dressing to check whether
blood is still oozing through. If it is do
not remove what you have put on for
this would disturb what clotting had
already occurred. Get or improvize
another pad and another bandage and
secure these over the first ones.

Keep the patient at rest. Cover him
to maintain his body temperature
(with blanket, coat, sacking). But do
not overheat (see p. 106). Let an
affected limb lie raised against something soft. Send for help.

Tourniquets are Forbidden

A tourniquet is a band wrapped very tightly round a limb in an attempt to reduce or arrest blood supply beyond it. However, unless skilfully applied from special bandages, it is likely to damage underlying structures including muscles and nerves. Also it carries the danger of being left on too long so that the extremity of the limb could be threatened by gangrene. *Tourniquets are not used in first aid.*

The only—and very rare—exception is the accidental amputation of a limb with heavy bleeding. In this case a tourniquet at the stump edge could be justified.

The Embedded Object

Do not remove anything stuck deeply in the wound. Control severe bleeding by pressing with a thumb on either side of the wound edge. (If you are without help you are now at a disadvantage since you have no free hand for other actions. You may have to try, instead of thumbs, pressing with the index and middle finger of one hand.)

Get thick pads banked round the wound, well above the level of the embedded object. Your tight bandage will then not push on it. A ring pad (see p. 17) could be very helpful here.

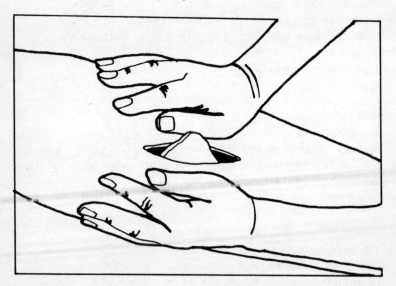

Pressure Points in Limbs

There are times when direct pressure on the severely bleeding wound of a limb will not serve. The cut may be so deep or the vessel so large that pressure fails. Or there may be so much additional damage to the area that pressure should not be attempted, as in a fracture with considerable bone splintering.

As an analogy imagine a kitchen sink with water flooding out from a burst pipe. A rug or towel could be forced against the break to stop the flow. If this does not work or if the broken pipe is inaccessible, then you have to turn off water at the mains.

In the same way if direct pressure cannot control bleeding the first aider will have to block the upper extremity of the artery which is bringing blood into the limb. He uses the *pressure point*, the spot at which this artery is just under the skin and also overlies a bone against which it can be compressed.

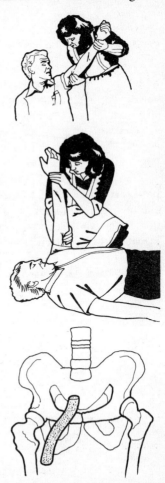

Arm Pressure Point

The artery runs on the inner side of the upper arm, along a line which corresponds to the inner seam of a sleeve.

Rapidly move behind your patient. With one hand on his wrist raise the arm. (If it may be fractured leave out this movement). At the same time cup your other hand under the upper part of the arm; curl your fingers and press with their tips. They will line over the artery and compress it down on the bone. If you do not succeed at once shift the finger positions slightly until you stop the bleeding. The pulse will also be blocked, which you can confirm by your hand at the wrist (see p. 25). As soon as possible lie the patient down.

Leg Pressure Point

The artery passes into the thigh at the line of the groin over the bony rim of the front of the pelvis. Quickly lie the patient down on his back and bend his knee (which relaxes the muscles). Press down immediately below the centre point of the groin. Quite a lot of pressure is needed, for the artery is big; use superimposed thumbs or (with extended arm) the heel of the hand or the closed fist.

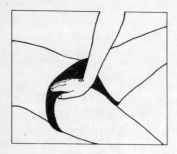
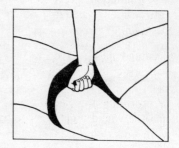

Pressure Point Risks

Use these two pressure points only when unavoidable in an emergency, when direct pressure on the wound is impossible. By blocking the artery you are cutting the blood supply not only from the bleeding point but also from the whole limb.

Maintain this pressure for no more than fifteen minutes, during which time raise your voice and call urgently for expert help. If help does not come by the end of that time very gently release your pressure without moving the limb. By now a clot may have formed and staunched the bleeding. If it has not you will have to reapply pressure for another fifteen minutes; but at least you will have allowed a brief blood flow to the whole limb to help keep its tissues alive. You may have to repeat this every fifteen minutes.

Bleeding from Particular Places

The Palm

Control immediately by grasping the patient's hand with your thumb

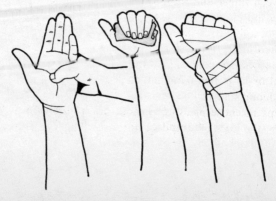

pressed on the wound. Keep it thus while you improvize a thick pad, and now let the patient clench it hard in his fist. Bandage over the hand firmly, leaving the thumb out. Keep the arm raised in a sling (see p. 18) or by pinning his sleeve cuff to the top of his jacket.

The Scalp

Bleeding could be heavy as the scalp has a copious blood supply, and also elastic fibres which tend to pull back and widen the wound when cut.

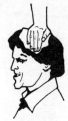

Controlling the bleeding is a problem if the wound might be accompanied by an underlying skull fracture (e.g. from a blow to the head). Unguarded pressure could worsen the bone damage. Do not use the tips of the fingers to press; keep the fingers together pressing evenly and widely over a big pad. If it can be managed, it is better to bandage firmly over a large ring pad (see p. 17) encompassing the area.

Nose Bleeding

Heavy nose bleeding can follow congestion from a cold or from raised blood pressure rupturing a small vessel. The bleeding point is inside the soft lower part of the nose.

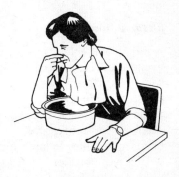

The patient must not sniff, blow his nose or push in pads, all of which would disturb clot formation.

He sits up, bending forwards and pinches the whole *lower* part of his nose between finger and thumb. Let him gently spit into a bowl any blood which might still be trickling down the back of the throat. It is best if he sits with his elbow on a table and wears a bib (towel or large handkerchief) to catch any blood stains.

He keeps the nose pressure without interruption for at least ten minutes (by the clock). If this does not succeed let him try another ten minutes.

Anyone above middle age who has had a sudden nose bleed, without obvious cause, could sensibly visit his doctor to request a check on his blood pressure.

Nose bleeding after injury to the head

This could be a more severe matter. A hard blow to the head may fracture the base of the skull, the bony 'shelf' on which the brain rests, and this might be revealed as nose bleeding (see p. 118).

Gum Bleeding

This nuisance can happen some hours after a tooth has been extracted. Do not let the patient keep on rinsing out his mouth for this would disturb clot formation. Exceptionally he could rinse just once to help to see clearly which socket is involved. Let the patient sit down and bite hard on a thick cloth (e.g. folded handkerchief) which is placed across the tooth socket (but not pressed down into it). The pad bridges over the hollow and allows clotting to form within the socket.

The patient keeps up the biting pressure for ten to twenty minutes. He will find it easier to manage if he sits with his elbow on the table and his hand cupped under the chin giving counter pressure. By tilting his head down, and to one side, the patient discharges any blood still oozing into the mouth.

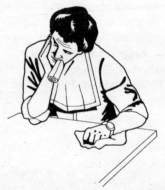

Bleeding from the Ear

A little blood and pus may come out of the ear after a day or so of intense earache. This could be due to an infection within the ear, in which pus under pressure has perforated the drum. With the release of pressure, as the discharge escapes, the pain is likely to subside. Do not put in any drops. Do not plug with wool; let the pus drain out. Apply a simple ear cover of clean cloth (gauze, folded handkerchief) kept on by bandage or adhesive tape, and consult a doctor.

However, the flow of blood or blood-tinged watery fluid which follows a blow to the head is quite different. This suggests a fracture of the skull where it overlies the ear canal. The amount of blood is not likely to be great; the danger lies in the possible damage to the brain. Also there is risk of infection reaching the brain, through the break,

from germs on the skin lining the ear
canal. Blood which clots in this canal
can act as nourishment to germs,
speeding their multiplication. In this
case therefore the blood should be
encouraged to flow out.

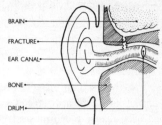

Lie the patient with the affected ear
pointing downwards. Cover the whole
outer ear with a clean cloth, kept on by adhesive strapping or
bandages. Do not plug the canal. Keep the patient quiet and call a
doctor.

If the patient is unconscious put him in the Recovery Position (see
p. 112) with the affected ear lower.

Coughing up Blood

Spots of blood produced by the strain of heavy coughing are not
dangerous in themselves. But they should never be ignored. Rarely
they can arise from a lung infection or a tumour. It is not only wise but
essential to get medical advice.

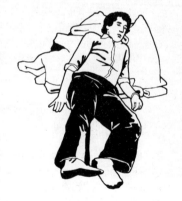

Larger amounts of blood coughed
up from the lungs will be bright red
and may be frothy, because they are
mixed with air. Lie the patient down
and get medical help urgently. Should
you know from which lung the blood
has come, make him lie on or towards
that side, for this will avoid any blood
coming up flowing backwards down
the air tube into the other lung. If his
breathing is difficult let him be also
half propped up (the 'semi-recumbent'
position) as this makes the chest
movements more effective. (See also
Chest Wounds, p. 51.)

Vomiting Blood

A blood vessel of the stomach lining may rupture from inflammation,
from an ulcer or from the effect of some drugs to which the patient has
the misfortune to be sensitive.

As a rule this bleeding is painless and gradual so that blood accumulates slowly within the stomach. Here it is acted on by digestive juices, which darken its colour. If the patient vomits now, he brings up brown or black material looking like coffee grounds. This may puzzle but not alarm him, but doctors, nurses and first aiders will know the significance.

Lie the patient down, preferably in the Recovery Position (see p. 112) and call a doctor. Give nothing by mouth.

Very rarely bleeding and vomit are so fast that there has been no time for the digestive action; the blood brought up is recognizably red. This needs full anti-shock care (see p. 105), urgent medical help and ambulance transport to hospital.

Hidden Internal Bleeding

This is specially dangerous as it does not show except by the deterioration of the patient's condition. Bleeding from an internal organ like a kidney, stomach or spleen could follow a severe blow or crush or could be due to infection or ulcer damaging a blood vessel. Blood can collect in a body cavity without showing up externally. (It might eventually appear as bruising or by passing out through the back passage or with the urine.)

Suspect hidden internal bleeding if the patient begins developing signs of shock (see p. 102). Lie him down, well covered, with head low and legs raised. Get immediate medical help or an ambulance to take him to hospital.

Questions

1. An elderly man interrupts his work because he feels sick. Soon after he vomits some slimy fluid mixed with dark brown matter. How would you help?

2. What is the disadvantage of using a pressure point, and how could you minimize this? What would make you decide to use a pressure point?

3. How would you describe the functions and importance of blood?

4. You are crossing a field with a friend. He trips over discarded machinery half hidden in the grass and gashes his thigh. As he picks himself up blood escapes freely from the wound. Describe in detail what you do.

5. An elderly man has been attended by his wife for copious bleeding from one nostril. After lying him down she put a cold wet cloth behind his neck, and pushed gauze into the nostril. Bleeding continues. What do you do? What advice do you give?

4
Lungs and Breathing

Mechanics of Breathing

Air breathed in contains oxygen, which passes into the blood (p. 24). Life processes in the body turn the oxygen into carbon dioxide. Then the blood stream brings the carbon dioxide to the lungs to be breathed out.

Whether one is awake and alert, or fast asleep the muscle movements, which control breathing, continue automatically.

1. The diaphragm, the large dome which acts as 'floor' to the chest or 'ceiling' to the abdominal cavity, tightens and flattens down, increasing the depth of the chest.

2. At the same time the small but powerful muscles running from rib to adjacent rib tighten and pull the ribs outwards.

In this double way the whole chest widens and air is drawn through the air passages from the back of the throat into the lungs whose elasticity allows them to expand. The muscles now relax, the chest contracts, the lungs narrow and air is pushed out.

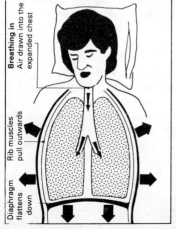
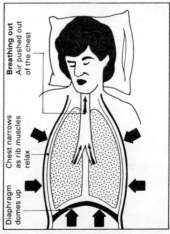

The Air Route

Air passes through the nose or mouth to the back of the throat and so into the windpipe.

Within the chest the windpipe divides into two main air tubes, one for each lung. Each then branches very many times into extremely fine tubes, which end up as clusters of minute air sacs. The air sacs are covered by a network of microscopically small blood vessels. It is here that oxygen passes from the lungs into the blood and carbon dioxide from the blood into the lungs.

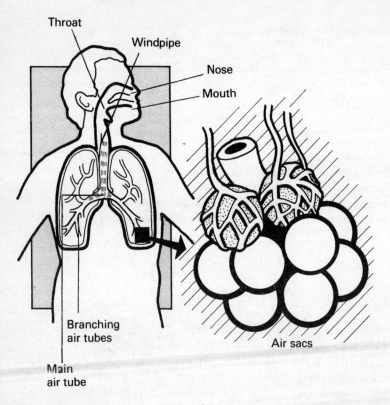

Throat

Windpipe

Nose

Mouth

Branching air tubes

Air sacs

Main air tube

The Breathing Rate

In a normal adult, at rest, this double movement varies from 12 to 18 times a minute. Children have a faster rate—from 24 to 40. The newborn baby may breathe about 50 to 60 times a minute. As with the pulse rate the breathing rate of the healthy adult can increase with exercise or emotion. The rate also rises in any condition where the body's oxygen needs are high or where there is difficulty in getting sufficient oxygen for ordinary tissue needs (e.g. fevers, lung illnesses, blood loss or asthma).

To count the breathing rate you simply watch the chest movements for 15 seconds and multiply the count by 4. Occasionally the shallowness of breathing or the bulk of the patient's coverings makes this difficult. But usually you can find some viewpoint, some prominent feature of clothing, which displays the chest's action. As with checking the pulse rate, experience counts and you should practice by unobtrusively watching the breathing of people at rest around you.

Breathing Difficulties and Asphyxia

Breathing may become handicapped in different ways.

1. *Illness of the lungs and air tubes* as in pneumonia and in asthma (p. 188).
2. *Failure of brain centres and nerves* which control breathing. Electrocution and some poisons can do this as well as certain forms of stroke, or a neck injury which damages the spinal cord.
3. *Damage to the chest or lung.* This includes wounds and blows, or a chest might be unable to move because of abnormal pressure on it as when someone is partly buried by a fall of sand.
4. *Poison in the air.* The most common example of this is the presence of carbon monoxide (p. 161).
5. *Obstruction to breathing. Suffocation* generally refers to an obstruction over the mouth and nose, but can also cover drowning or breathing air with heavy fumes, or with very little oxygen.

Choking describes obstruction in the air passage itself, at the back of the throat or in the windpipe. It could also be the result of hanging or strangling. For an unconscious man his own tongue might create the danger: this is described on p. 49.

Asphyxia is the word which sums up the worst consequences of all these conditions. Its medical meaning is the situation where body tissues are dangerously starved of oxygen. But custom has narrowed the definition to lack of air in the lungs. The brain, with its many centres controlling life maintenance, is far more critically sensitive to lack of oxygen than is any other organ. Thus sustained asphyxia can lead to brain failure, and brain failure to cessation of breathing efforts and of heart beats. *In all cases, once you have coped with the airway obstruction, check whether the patient is breathing. If he is not begin resuscitation at once* (p. 130).

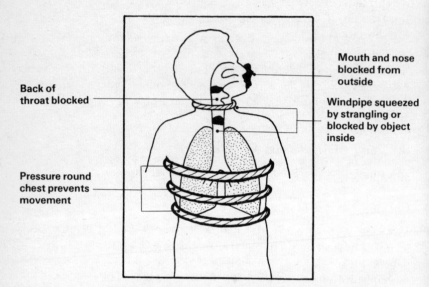

Back of throat blocked

Mouth and nose blocked from outside

Windpipe squeezed by strangling or blocked by object inside

Pressure round chest prevents movement

The airway can be obstructed at many points.

Hanging

Although often suicidal, hanging, by cord or wire, can be accidental as with children throttled by anorak hood cords or by climbing frames.

Support the victim by the legs to relieve the tension and cut the cord. Be prepared to catch the weight of the body as it is released. Ease the tight band at the neck, or cut the cord, which may be deeply set in its own groove.

Strangling

This may result from accident. A scarf or necktie caught in machinery could have been pulled tight round the neck.

Deal with this as for hanging except that you do not have to support the weight of the victim's body.

Suffocation

The rescue of someone in a room filled with fumes or dangerous gases is as for those in a smoke-laden atmosphere (see p. 92). A baby may be smothered by a soft pillow or a child by the plastic bag he has pulled over his face.

Alternatively the victim may be an adult caught in an atmosphere whose oxygen supply has been used up: this can happen where a fire burns a long time in a room where ventilation is poor and fresh air does not enter. First remove the patient from the injurious atmosphere, or the covering from the patient.

If someone has been buried under a fall of earth or snow you will clear more than his face before beginning artificial respiration. Get his chest free of the weight upon it so that it can expand with the breathing attempts.

Choking

The back of the throat or the windpipe can be blocked by displaced dentures, by food, vomit or blood or by a sucked-in toy. Generally the patient will be coughing or making harsh breathing noises as he tries to overcome this. If air to his lungs is severely limited his face becomes pale, then blue and soon he may collapse unconscious.

A quick but careful scoop with your forefinger might hook the obstruction away from the back of the throat. Curve the finger and reach the offending object by moving carefully sideways along the inside of the cheek. Remember that you aim to give a forward movement with your finger tip and that you must avoid pushing the object further back.

But do not spend too much time and effort using your finger. In most cases the obstructing object is beyond reach. It blocks the windpipe partly or completely. The situation can be worsened by the way the obstructing object is held more firmly as the windpipe tightens up from irritation and also from its reflex reaction to the patient's fright.

The choking patient begins to cough. As long as some air can get in and out, coughing and speaking is possible. But if obstruction is total he cannot expel air to cough or to speak. Do not disregard the silent victim struggling with his hands at his throat. That he is not coughing should alarm and alert rather than reassure you. Ask him clearly if he is choking; he may be able to answer by nodding his head.

The man who deliberately or automatically puts a hand up, to the front of his neck, with thumb on one side and fingers on the other, is making the signal which indicates 'Help me—I am choking'.

Give help in the stages described below according to the state of the patient. After each step be prepared to examine the mouth and to use your fingers to hook out quickly the obstructing object which has been brought up but which is still lying in the mouth; do not let the patient breathe it back.

1. The Alert, Active, Coughing and Spluttering Patient

Blockage is partial. His coughing is a healthy reflex and you do not interfere but you watch closely. Do not let the patient leave the room unattended. You can advise him to breathe slowly and deeply as this might help to reduce the tight spasm of the windpipe. Also let him try separate deliberate and heavy coughs instead of a great number of smaller, irregular ones.

2. The Patient Cannot Manage to Cough Strongly or is Silent

No longer does he seem in control. Coughing is weakening. Or there may be no noise as blockage is complete. He cannot speak.

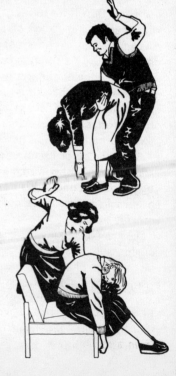

Give Blows to the Back

They aim to shake and dislodge the obstructing object. Bend the patient forward with his head as low as possible. A child you can hold over your forearm or on your bent knee with his head down. A very small child you can also hold—very firmly—upside down by his ankles.

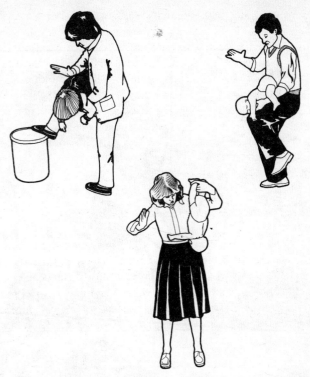

If an adult has fallen to the ground, kneel by him. Bend his head well back, turn him on his side, his chest resting on your thighs and slap the back.

With the heel of your hand give a *really hard* blow between the shoulder blades. If this does not succeed try it again up to three more times before moving on to:

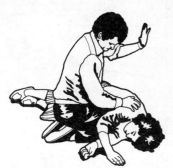

Abdominal Thrusts

By compressing the abdomen below the diaphragm these thrusts aim to increase chest pressure and propel the object out, rather like a pea from a pea shooter.

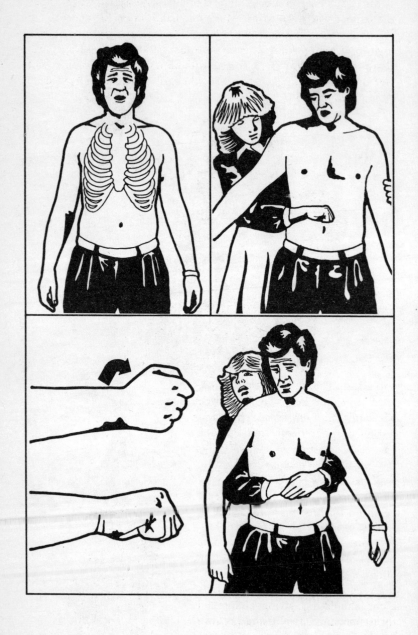

Move behind the patient and make him bend well down. Encircle the patient with your arms. Make one hand into a fist and place it *thumb end first* in a position *half-way between the lower end of the breastbone and the navel.* Cup your other hand over it. Give a hard, sharp thrust *inwards and upwards* with both your hands. You do not give the thrust by hugging (which could harm the ribs) but by sharply bending your elbows.

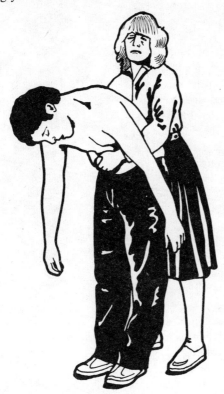

You can do abdominal thrusts to someone who is sitting by getting behind his chair. Indeed this position allows a child to act on an adult.

(A choking person who is quite alone should try giving abdominal thrusts to himself by using his own hands. Or he could do it by thrusting his upper abdomen very hard against

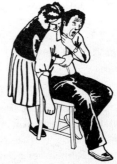

a suitable horizontal bar like a railing or the upper edge of a chair back. He should keep his windpipe straight by holding his chin up.)

If the patient is on the ground make him lie on his back with his head bent back. Kneel across him with a leg on either side of his hips. (Merely kneeling at one side would give badly directed pressure.) Put the heel of one hand on the abdomen in the position described above, place the other hand over it and give the thrust this way.

A child is treated in the same manner except that the thrust is less forceful. You can sit the child on your lap, with his back against your chest. A baby you place on his back or you hold him firmly with his back on your forearm which you rest on your bent thigh. Give the thrust with only a couple of fingers.

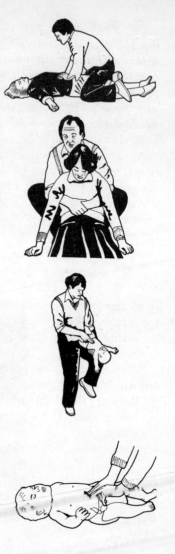

With a successful thrust the object may be blown up into the mouth (whence you will quickly retrieve it) or it may shoot out of the mouth with some force.

If the thrust does not succeed repeat, up to three more times. If this fails now repeat, alternately, the attempts by back blows and by abdominal thrusts (four attempts each) until either you succeed or the patient becomes unconscious.

3. If the Patient Becomes Unconscious, No Longer Making Breathing Attempts

You begin artificial ventilation at once (p. 131). The windpipe is likely to have relaxed when the patient lost consciousness. As you give artificial ventilation you may find that the air you breathe into the patient can slip past the obstruction. It is not likely to blow the object deeper in. Remember how important it is to have his head bent well back, his nose pinched and your mouth properly positioned (pp. 132–3).

However you could find that, even with accurate technique, you cannot get air into the patient and that his chest does not rise because the obstruction persists. Then you must continue to try to dislodge it with back blows and with abdominal thrusts as already described. This will, of course, involve repeatedly turning him on his side (for the back blows) and on his back (for the abdominal thrusts).

After each of the series of four blows and that of four thrusts you should probe the mouth with your curved forefinger to see if the object has come up and is lying by the throat ready to be hooked out.

And after each set of abdominal thrusts again try if artificial ventilation is now possible. The chart below shows how you continue the cycle of ventilation attempts, of back blows and of abdominal thrusts as long as may be necessary.

Important

In all cases, where you have given abdominal thrusts make sure that the patient is medically checked immediately afterwards. The thrust, a life-saving measure, carries a small risk of doing some internal damage.

Also once an unconscious patient, to whom you have given artificial ventilation recovers his spontaneous breathing, you should put him in the Recovery Position (p. 112). Watch him closely in case he stops and needs help again. Get him to hospital by ambulance.

Finally: when learning, never practice the full thrust or the ventilation on a volunteer. Practice only on a manikin.

Postscript on First Aid for Choking

It is clear that there are two different ways of trying to clear an obstructing object from the windpipe.

1. Back slaps to loosen the grip of the windpipe and dislodge the object so that it can be expelled. This method has been taught for very many years.

2. Abdominal thrusts to force air up the windpipe and, with it, the obstructing object. This is a relatively recent method.

Back slaps are quick and easy to give. The important point is that *the patient must have chest and head pointing well down.* Otherwise, by simple gravity, the dislodged object could slip deeper down and worsen the situation. With the abdominal thrust, which is almost as easy, the patient's position is less significant.

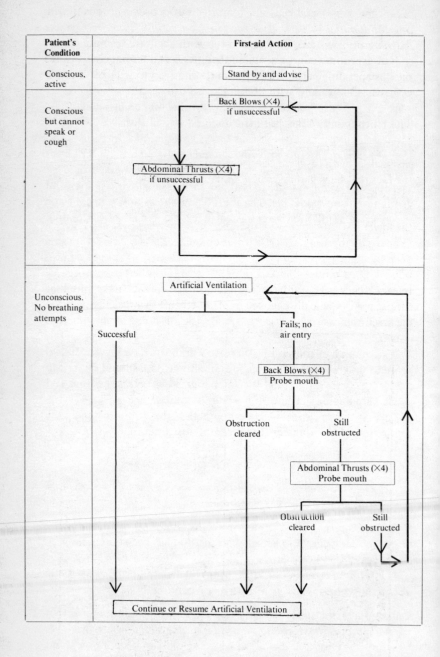

Patient's Condition	First-aid Action
Conscious, active	Stand by and advise
Conscious but cannot speak or cough	Back Blows (×4) if unsuccessful → Abdominal Thrusts (×4) if unsuccessful
Unconscious. No breathing attempts	Artificial Ventilation — Successful / Fails; no air entry → Back Blows (×4) Probe mouth → Obstruction cleared / Still obstructed → Abdominal Thrusts (×4) Probe mouth → Obstruction cleared / Still obstructed → Continue or Resume Artificial Ventilation

So there is a very strong case for omitting the back slaps and trying only abdominal thrusts. And therefore an equally good reason for teaching only the latter method.

However these pages have described the use of both methods since back slaps still feature in many authoritatively-organized first-aid courses.

The Unconscious Man and his Tongue

If at any time you discover someone who is unconscious and lying on his back or with his head bent forward, you must take very seriously the fact that he is in danger of choking because of the blocking action of his tongue.

The tongue is a muscle which is attached by its base to the sides of the lower jaw-bone with its front free. In a conscious person (A) or in a sleeper (B) the tongue, like all muscles, has its own natural tension keeping it in place. But if someone is unconscious due to illness, poisoning or injury, then his muscles, including the tongue, become relaxed. The tongue will tend to flop back against the throat, blocking the airway (C). Unfortunately many deaths from asphyxia have occurred this way.

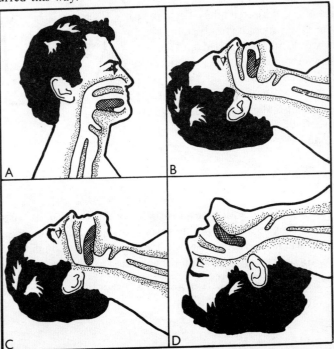

The remedy is simple. By gently bending the head back as far as it will go you move the tongue from the back of the throat and you re-open the airway (D).

This manoeuvre may look slight, but it can be life-saving. Once you have done it you must keep the head in this position until the patient regains consciousness. You will never raise his head on a pillow. See the chapter on unconsciousness (p. 110) for further details.

Chest Injuries

Bleeding within Lungs and Airways

Because it is mixed with air any blood coughed up is likely to be bright red and frothy. If bleeding is severe it is possible that some blood spills over from the main air tube of the injured side into that of the other side at the point where the two join. Since the flow will follow the law of gravity this would mean blood entering the airways of the uninjured lung. Were you to turn the patient on to his good side you would increase this risk. Therefore you should keep the uninjured side uppermost and lie the patient on or towards the injured side. This position also allows the good lung to move freely unimpeded by pressure and do the work for both.

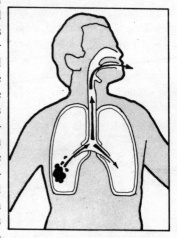

Blast Injury

A strong air blast of an explosion can so compress the chest wall that it destroys lung tissue without however showing outward injuries. The patient will have great breathing difficulties. He may cough up blood. This can happen also to a swimmer subjected to the pressure caused by an underwater explosion.

The Open Chest Wound

An injury penetrating the chest can reach the underlying lung. Even if it goes no further than making a hole in the chest wall it can cause very serious trouble. With each inspiration taken by the patient air will not only enter the lungs through the mouth and air tubes, but also will be sucked into the chest space through the wound.

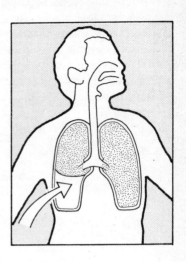

One could expect that, as the patient breathes out, this air, filling the chest space, will be expelled. However flaps of damaged tissue at the wound edges often act as valves; they open to admit air at inspiration but at expiration they close up and trap the air. With each breath more and more air builds up in the chest space around the lung, compressing and handicapping it. Eventually it may embarrass the heart's movements and those of the lung on the uninjured side.

It is urgently necessary to close the wound and make it as airtight as possible.

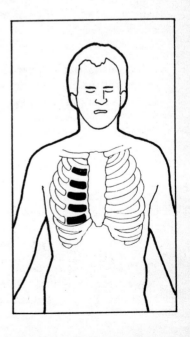

The Smashed Chest Wall

The term 'stove-in-chest' covers the type of injury where crushing or a wide blow fractures several ribs and perhaps also the breast bone. A whole area of the bony components of the chest wall breaks free from its normal attachments.

It now moves independently of the rest of the chest action, and it moves paradoxically. As the patient breathes out, this area can be seen to bulge forwards, while the rest of the chest contracts normally. It will also sink in while the rest of the chest expands during inspiration.

The mechanics of breathing are damaged; the lungs do not act properly and the patient cannot easily cough up any obstruction from his air passages.

First Aid to Chest Injuries

1. Ensure a clear airway

Quickly clear any obstructions such as loosened teeth, dentures, blood or vomit from the back of the mouth.

2. Close up any wound

Pinch its edges together or gently but firmly place the palm of your hand flat over the wound. You aim to make an airtight seal over it. Keep your hand in position until you have improvised and replaced your hand with a thick pad. Secure it firmly with wide bandages. Ideal seals would be covers of metal foil or thin plastic held by overlapping strips of adhesive strapping, if you have these to hand. But the strapping does not hold closely on a moist, perhaps bloodstained or hairy chest wall or over breasts.

3. Immobilize any unstable part

If you see the irregular 'paradoxical' movements of a stove-in-chest try to control the chest at once. Press the flat of your hand firmly but gently over it. As soon as possible replace your hand by a thick pad, well-bandaged or strapped down.

Put the arm of the injured side upwards across the chest in an elevation sling (p. 19) since this position can reduce the patient's suffering. In fact you can augment the pressure on the front of the chest by having the patient's arm (if it is uninjured) lying over the pad and under the bandaging. Pressure on an area at the back or side of the chest can be increased by letting the patient lie on this area.

4. Careful positioning

Position the patient with breathing difficulties by compromising between the needs of countering shock (p. 105) and those of easing his breathing. Put the *conscious* patient in what is called the 'semi-prone'

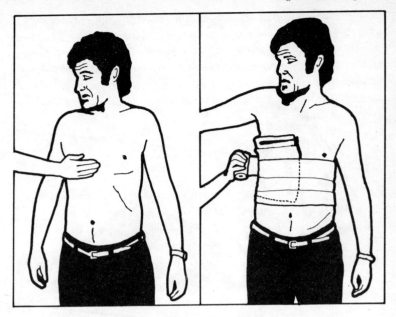

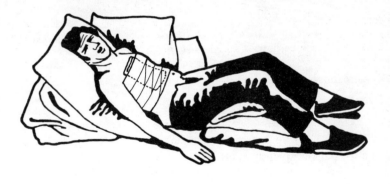

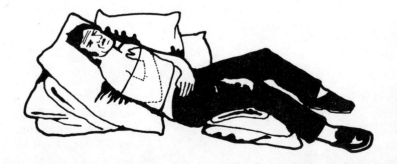

position, which is half-leaning and half-sitting. Bank him thus with pillows, folded coats or blankets. As you tend the patient's wound you can already help him into the right position by kneeling behind him so that your thigh supports his back and his head is cushioned by your abdomen or your chest.

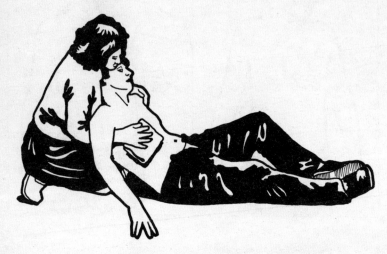

If he is *unconscious* place him in the Recovery Position (p. 112). In either case lie him *on or towards his injured side.*

5. *Anti-shock measures*

Give these as far as is possible (p. 105).

6. *Hospitalization*

Send the patient urgently to hospital.

Questions

1. A stranger suddenly chokes severely in a snack bar. With a few abdominal thrust attempts you manage to get him clear and breathing easily. After suitable expressions of gratitude he turns to go. Can you congratulate yourself on having completed the task?

2. 'For an unconscious man the most dangerous thing is his own tongue.' How can this be so? How would you overcome the danger.

3. What do you understand by asphyxia? Describe circumstances which might give rise to asphyxia.

4. In an explosion the left side of a man's chest is pierced by a fragment of metal which he immediately pulls out. He is coughing and breathless. How do you help?

5. At a dinner party one of your number splutters, coughs harshly once or twice and then silently makes for the door. Outline your actions.

5
Joints and Muscles

Movement and Stability

The firmness of the body is due primarily to internal stiffening by bones, with the assistance of muscles.

As well as determining a person's stature, stance and stability, many bones play a big protecting role. A study of the picture opposite shows some clear examples. Bones also have another and more subtle role, for it is in their marrow that blood cells are produced. Some of the anatomical names of bones are given for reference. You need not learn them for first aid unless taking a special course which requires this knowledge.

Joints

Bones link together at joints. Some of these are fixed and immovable. Most joints however allow movement of varying type.

Immovable

Those, with the bones fitting into each other closely and firmly, like those at the top of the skull, are immovable.

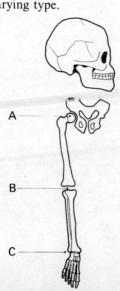

Movable

(A) *Ball and Socket.* The round end of one bone fits into the cup-like hollow of another, to give movement in many directions, e.g. the shoulder and the hip.

(B) *Hinge.* The end of one bone lies against the end of another, allowing bending and straightening in one

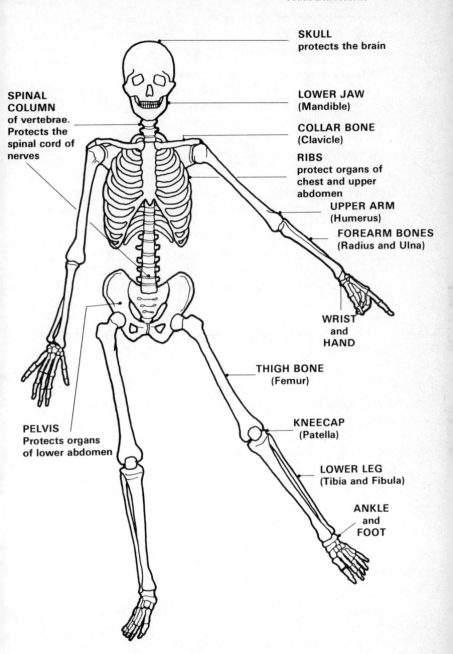

SKULL
protects the brain

LOWER JAW
(Mandible)

SPINAL COLUMN
of vertebrae.
Protects the
spinal cord of
nerves

COLLAR BONE
(Clavicle)

RIBS
protect organs of
chest and upper
abdomen

UPPER ARM
(Humerus)

FOREARM BONES
(Radius and Ulna)

WRIST
and
HAND

THIGH BONE
(Femur)

KNEECAP
(Patella)

PELVIS
Protects organs
of lower abdomen

LOWER LEG
(Tibia and Fibula)

ANKLE
and
FOOT

direction only: e.g. the elbow and the knee.

(C) *Slightly movable only* where stability is important: e.g. the ankle or between the bones of the vertebral column.

At these movable joints strong bands called *ligaments* hold the bones in place. The shape of the bones and the way they fit together limits the range of joint movement and to some extent so do the attachment and strength of the ligaments.

Muscles

Activating joints is the task of muscles. At each of their ends muscles are attached by strong bands (tendons) to the bones they serve. Controlled by nerves muscles can contract; becoming shorter and thicker they provide the pull and power for moving the bones.

In addition a muscle which creates one type of action (such as bending a limb) must be able to co-ordinate with a muscle which produces the opposite action (straightening the limb). As the one muscle contracts, so its opposite should relax. If both of them are partly and equally contracted, this combined tension keeps the limb position stable.

In the illustration bones of the leg are shown as solid lines and muscles as dotted lines.

Right Leg

To bend : 'A' contracts, pulling the lower leg up and back and bending the knee. At the same time 'B' relaxes and stretches to allow this movement.

To straighten and kick : 'B' contracts, pulling the knee straight and the leg forward. At the same time 'A' relaxes.

Left Leg

All this while both 'A' and 'B' are held in contraction to keep the leg firmly straight and upright.

Injuries to this system for which you may have to give first aid could include:

the muscles	:	strains and cramps;
the joints	:	sprains and (p. 90) dislocations;
the bones	:	fractures (p. 64);
the nerve system	:	strokes (p. 193).

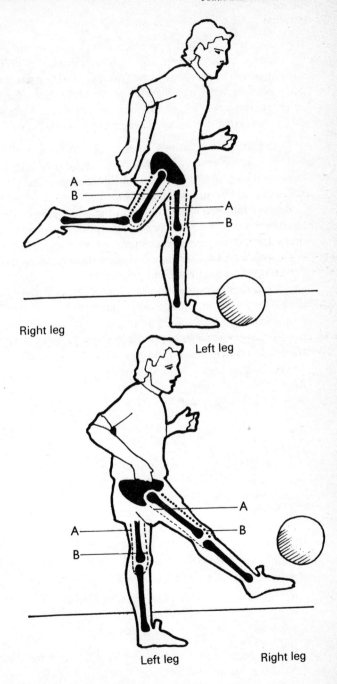

Right leg

Left leg

A

B

A

B

A

B

A

B

Left leg

Right leg

Strains

Do not confuse this with sprains (p. 61). A muscle can be strained by the overstretching or tearing of some of its fibres. This can happen by sudden severe exertion or in handling very heavy weights. It causes pain which is worsened by attempts to move. Sometimes, in severe cases, there is swelling or bruising. Be careful: if there has been an actual blow to the patient he may have sustained a fracture.

1. Let the patient adopts his most comfortable position.
2. If you see him within about half an hour of his injury, apply a cold compress (p. 62). By its cooling action it reduces the blood flow in the area and this limits the swelling.

But by about thirty minutes after the injury the swelling is likely to have become complete. From this point of view there would be small point in beginning the cold compress at this relatively late stage. Yet it is possible that the cold might slightly relieve the patient's pain.

3. The main treatment is to put the part at rest and to support it. If it is a limb apply an elastic or a crêpe bandage firmly over thick padding.

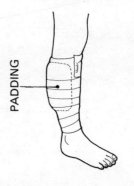

Take care not to make it so tight as to obstruct the circulation. Also avoid extending it to cover a joint like ankle, knee, wrist or elbow: at these sites nerves and blood vessels lie very close to the skin surface and may be subjected to undue pressure by the bandage.

Warn the patient to report at once if the limb beyond the bandage becomes cold, numb, blue, white or puffy: the pressure of the bandage might need to be reduced.

If the arm or hand is involved have it supported in a sling (p. 18).

Cramps

Cramps are sudden involuntary sustained contractions of muscles. They may be strong enough to be very painful. Very often this can be 'switched off' by strongly stretching the cramped muscle as far as it will go.

Cramp in the calf

Sit the patient down and straighten his knee; then bend the foot upwards as far as possible.

Cramp at the back of thigh

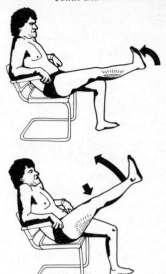

Sit the patient down and straighten his knee. Raise his leg by the heel as far as possible; at the same time put one hand over the front of the knee and press firmly down here.

Where it is not practicable to stretch the muscle, you may be able to give the patient good relief by massaging the area with deep firm pressure.

Sometimes generalized cramp can hit a person whose body has become depleted of minerals and fluids. This could happen fairly suddenly after severe diarrhoea and vomiting or excessive sweating. Your treatment is to restore the missing items. Give the patient water to which you have added a teaspoonful of salt in each litre (approximately two pints). Alternatively he can drink a weak preparation of meat or vegetable extracts. Give it tepid rather than hot, and advise him to drink it in slow sips. Fast drinking could worsen any vomiting or diarrhoea.

Sprains

Do not confuse these with strains (p. 60).

In a sprain a joint has been forcibly overstretched. The main damage is tearing fibres of the ligaments, which secure the bones at the joint. The most common example is the sprained ankle as the foot accidentally and sharply turns in, pulling on the ligaments over the outer side of the ankle.

Be careful to suspect a fracture (p. 68) if the patient received a blow at the joint. Occasionally a very sharp twist of the foot and its ligaments actually makes the ligament pull so hard that it breaks off a small fragment of bone from the lower end of the outer leg bone; the patient is likely to have felt a 'snap' as it happened.

Treatment of sprains is as for strains (p. 60) with a cold compress and firm support. The difference here is that your supporting bandage and padding will go over the joint. At most joints, nerves and blood vessels lie close to the surface so you must be very careful to avoid undue pressure, especially in the hollow of the knee or the bend of the elbow. Use thick padding like cotton wool to cover the joint and the area on each side of it; then apply the supporting bandage over it and between each of its first two turns interleave more padding. This evens out the pressure without weakening it.

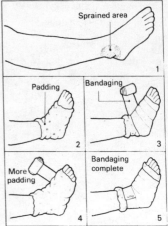

The Cold Compress

Soak a piece of thick material like flannel or a small towel in cold water. If you have ice cubes add a few to the water. Wring out excess water, so that it remains wet but not dripping. Fold it to the size needed and lay it over the injured area. To be effective it should not warm up. If you have to use something to hold it in position use very light open-weave material like gauze, or thin bandage strips round the edges. Keep the compress in position for about half an hour. Should it dry, drip a little more cold water on it.

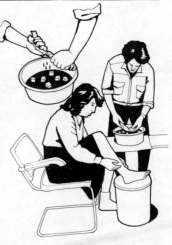

Hernia

Muscles which form the wall over the front of the abdomen are subject to all sorts of strains. Heavy lifting and pulling or even hard coughing may separate some of their fibres. Then the tension within the abdomen could make some part of the abdominal contents protrude, showing as a soft lump under the skin. This is a hernia or 'rupture'. What protrudes can be a fold of the membranes which lie within the abdomen and often also, tucked in this fold, a short length of bowel.

Of the several places where this can happen the most common are at the groin (A) and by the navel (B). Sometimes an abdominal operation leaves a weakened muscle so that a hernia could occur in the scar region (C).

As the rupture happens the patient may feel a sudden, momentary, pain and soon after he discovers the lump. Quite often the bulge shows when he is standing but by gravity flattens and disappears if he lies down.

Hernias are rarely first-aid problems. In due course the patient will consult his doctor who will advise on treatment (generally a surgical repair). Occasionally however the pain or discomfort is intense and continuing. Also it could happen that the parts which have protruded become twisted and compressed, impeding their blood supply and threatening gangrene. The lump becomes firmer and tender.

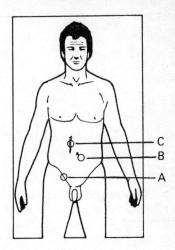

If you are called upon to help someone whose hernia is giving distress do **not** try to push the lump back. The tissues are inflamed and the pathway of the protrusion is not always a straight one; pressure could be harmful. Aim to reduce the compression on the hernia by relaxing the muscles involved. Let the patient lie down with his knees bent over some support like a pillow and with his head and shoulders comfortably raised. This position is similar to that used in the case of abdominal wounds (p. 4). Then get medical advice quickly.

Questions

1. A friend telephones to ask advice about her husband who has just sprained his elbow lifting a heavy sack. What detailed instructions would you give her?

2. You wake in the middle of the night with painful cramp in the calf. How do you cope?

3. What is the difference between a sprain and a strain? Is there any difference in their treatment?

4. You are helping a friend move heavy paving stones in his garden. He drops his load and complains of a sharp strain at the top of one leg. After about an hour's rest he is still in pain. You find a small, fairly firm and very tender bulging of the skin near his groin. What is your advice?

5. Describe five different organs in the body which are protected, fully or partly, by bones. Give the simple names of these bones.

6
Fractures: General Principles

A broken bone has a natural tendency to heal. If the damaged ends are close to each other new soft tissue grows to bridge the gap. In time hard bony substance forms within the softness and a rigid repair takes place.

Difficulties would arise had the broken ends been displaced relatively far from each other, or had there been much damage to the area around the bone, especially if the blood supply had been weakened. Sometimes the broken bone ends cut into important organs. Another type of interference would be infection which can interfere with bone repair. All these can have happened at the moment of fracture, and this will give the doctors extra work and the patient extra distress.

Also such mishaps can be caused, or worsened, by well-meaning but careless or ignorant people who come to help. As a first aider you will use caution and your special knowledge to protect the patient.

This chapter describes the general principles of how fractures happen, are diagnosed and are given first aid. The next chapter applies these principles to the fracture of specific bones, detailing methods which experience has shown to be best. You should learn and practice them. *But you must be absolutely certain about the general principles.* They are simple and straightforward. Even if you forget the detailed teaching for any individual bone, your memory of the principles will prevent you from going wrong.

How a Fracture Happens

A bone can be broken 'directly' or 'indirectly'.

Direct Fracture

The break occurs where the blow falls. Examples are many: a leg run over by a car wheel; a hammer blow on a finger; a wrist bone broken by someone falling on it; a heel bone broken by a high jump on to a hard surface; a skull hit by a falling object.

Indirect Fracture

Less obviously this happens when a bone breaks some distance from the site of the blow, the force having been transmitted through other bones. A hard blow on the head may crack the base of the skull (that inner 'shelf' on which the brain rests); someone falling on the lower part of the leg could break the upper end of the thigh bone, where it is angled to form a joint with the socket in the pelvis; a fall on the outstretched arm can carry a jerk to the shoulder, sharply levering up and snapping the collar bone.

You must remember the way these forces can move, so that you do not overlook the indirect fractures they may cause.

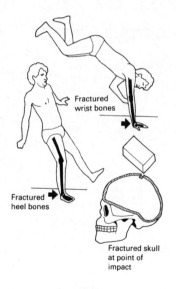

Fractured wrist bones

Fractured heel bones

Fractured skull at point of impact

DIRECT

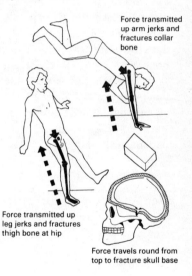

Force transmitted up arm jerks and fractures collar bone

Force transmitted up leg jerks and fractures thigh bone at hip

Force travels round from top to fracture skull base

INDIRECT

Closed and Open Fractures

As long as the skin is undamaged it acts as a relatively tough and thick shield against invasion by microbes from outside. A *closed fracture* is one in which the break is thus protected.

However the accident may break

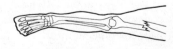

the skin so that the bone becomes
exposed to microbes. This is the *open
fracture*, with the risk of infection
which could delay or prevent bone
repair.

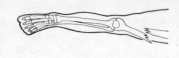

An open fracture is obvious when a
bit of bone protrudes from the skin or
is seen in the base of a large wound.
The open fracture could be almost
hidden when there is a narrow wound
track leading to the tissue depths in
which the broken bone lies; a bullet or
similar projectile could do this, as
could a very thin hard-pointed object.
First aid to open fractures begins with
careful dressing of the wound.

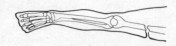

Bear in mind also the possibility of
the closed fracture with a displaced
bone end lying closely against the
skin. Mishandling could allow the
bone to move and pierce the skin. The
closed has now become an open
fracture—a great disservice to the
patient.

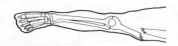

The Complicated Fracture

One cannot sustain a fracture
without, to some extent, involving
what lies near the bone. In this respect
any fracture is always complicated by
some bruising and by some damage to
neighbouring tissues. But the term
Complicated Fracture is used when a
really important organ is injured,
such as the severing of a major artery
or nerve.

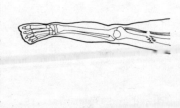

The illustration opposite shows the main possibilities of severe
complications at different points of the body. These disasters may
happen at the moment of the accident. But again they could be created
by the bone's shifting after the event, either because the victim has not
been still, or because the rescuer has been clumsy in his manipulations.

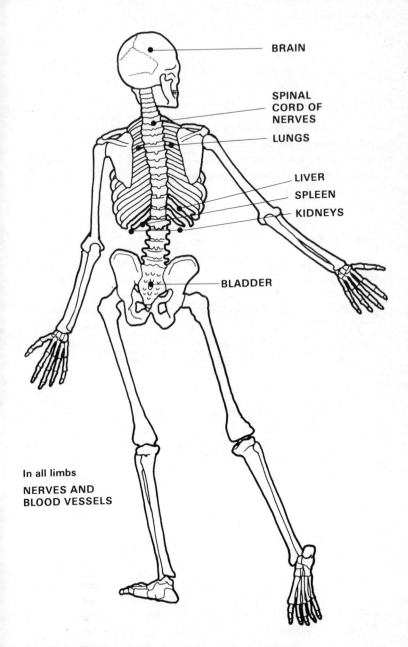

In all limbs
**NERVES AND
BLOOD VESSELS**

COMPLICATED FRACTURES: Possible organ damage at various sites

Remember

The important lesson is that fractures can often be much more than just a broken bone. First aid is likely to involve stopping severe bleeding and protecting any wounds as well as safeguarding the immobility of the injured part.

Diagnosing a Fracture

How does one know when a bone is fractured? Sometimes the diagnosis is only too clear as when a limb alignment is greatly deformed or if a bone protrudes. However in many cases it is a matter of uncertainty and even experienced doctors would need X-ray examinations to make sure.

Three features will make you suspect a fracture.

1. The History

The victim has received a heavy blow or bang; he may have had a severe wrench as could happen to a sharply twisted ankle; he could actually have felt the bone snap.

This is straightforward. Yet there are times when a severe impact has spared the bone. Others, more problematic, are when an apparently trivial knock has caused a fracture. The latter is more likely to happen to some elderly people with brittle bones.

2. The Symptoms

This word covers what the patient feels. *Pain* is the first symptom; its degree can be very variable and no true guide to the severity of the fracture. Then the patient is handicapped by *loss of power* in the affected part. For instance with a fractured wrist (and irrespective of the amount of pain) his hand movements and finger grip will be weakened. In addition there will be *loss of function*; he may not be able to get the wrist to move through its full range, even weakly.

Ideally, of course, no one should try to move a part which could be fractured. Unfortunately many patients do so immediately after the accident as a test of their state, which is thereby worsened.

3. The Signs

There are features which doctor, nurse or first aider discovers on careful examinations. And, often, so does the patient.

Swelling and *bruising* in the injured area are very likely. However swelling may not develop until some minutes after the accident. Bruising does not always happen and may not show up until even later—a matter of several hours.

Deformity is not always present. It shows if one part of the broken bone has become markedly displaced. The area may be irregular and unusually shaped; compare it with the corresponding area on the other side. In the skull there may be a depression, though this can rapidly become hidden by swelling of the overlying skin. A limb may look abnormally angled or twisted. Sometimes it appears a little shorter than that on the other side, as muscle spasm

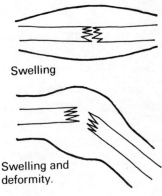

Swelling

Swelling and deformity.

displaces broken bone. Also there will be *tenderness*, i.e. pain caused by cautiously light touch. On no account should you go further and test movement of the injured part. This would be against all principles of first-aid protection.

Surveying these diagnostic points it seems that it could be very difficult to make up one's mind. Blows, weakness, reduced function, pain, swelling, and bruising, could be present after injuries like contusions, sprains, and strains. The only absolute initial evidence of a fracture would be marked deformity or the unfortunate sighting of a broken bone end in an open wound.

Do not let this discourage you. Your line of thought and action is simple:

> *If the circumstances suggest that*
> *there might be a fracture, treat*
> *the condition as a fracture.*

Subsequent examination by experts or by X-rays may show the bone to be intact, but you should then receive only praise for your caution. On the other hand you could well be blamed for inadequate attention to a fracture because you had thought that the history, symptoms, and signs were not severe enough.

> *Wherever there is doubt, the injury*
> *is guilty of being a fracture until*
> *investigations prove it to be innocent.*

Please note that this does not absolve you from carefully obtaining the history, asking about symptoms and examining for signs after the accident.

Treatment of Fractures: General Principles

The rules are extremely simple.

1. Warn the Patient not to Move

Warn bystanders also not to move him. The general tendency of the patient is to try to be active, and solicitous, but uninformed bystanders, tend to pick up a fallen victim.

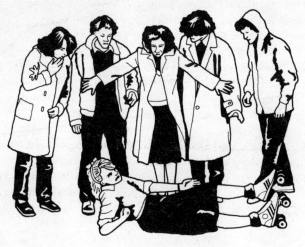

2. Stop any Severe Bleeding at Once (p. 27)

Try to do this without moving the part suspected to be fractured.

If you do move it be as gentle as possible. Regard the necessary movement as the lesser of two evils. Uncontrolled heavy bleeding would be by far the greater danger to the patient.

3. Dress any Wound (p. 2)

Here again try to avoid moving the fracture area. Even a hastily improvized clean cover is important to minimize contamination by microbes. If a broken bone end projects from a wound, dress this as you would a wound with an embedded object (p. 4).

It may seem that so far you have done nothing specific for the fracture itself but already you have achieved a lot. You have protected the patient against blood loss and against infection. And by his immobility you have made sure that the broken bone ends do not become more displaced and do no further tissue and organ damage around them.

4. *Immobilize the Fracture*

(If however you expect medical or ambulance help to be quickly available it may be wise to do no more and to leave it to the experts.)

You immobilize by applying a splint. In some cases you can improvize a splint out of slabs of wood, cardboard or even magazines. A magazine or thick newspaper, rolled up and tied, then padded and bandaged, makes an improvized splint on which to immobilize a forearm, elbow, and wrist.

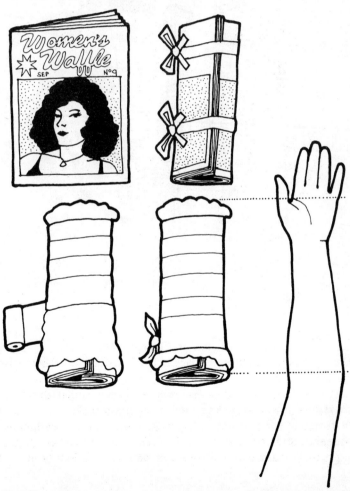

But for the majority of fractures, the best and ever present split is the patient's own body; injured arm is splinted by the chest or injured leg splinted by the good leg.

The diagrams below illustrate the principles to follow.

(A) Do not remove clothing unless this is absolutely necessary. Sometimes you may have to cut the clothing, but spare it, if you can.

(B) Avoid as far as possible moving the injured part.

(C) Move the uninjured part (e.g. the good leg) up against the injured part.

(D) Plan immobilization to include not only the whole of the broken bone but also any joint at either end.

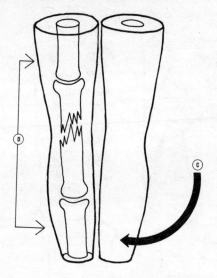

(E) Put padding (e.g. scarves, wool, socks, folded towels) fitting fully (not loosely) in hollows between the body parts to give stability, and also between adjacent bumps to prevent rubbing.

(F) Bandage the two parts firmly enough to prevent any movement. If an injured limb is lying on the ground do not lift it to fit the bandage. Slip the bandage under a natural hollow and then gently slide it to the required level. Place all bandages in position before tying them

(G) But put no bandage over the area of the suspected fracture.

(H) Tie the bandage knots on the uninjured side.

Throughout any handling, steady and support the injured part until immobilization is completed. If you cannot avoid moving a fractured limb, move it as a whole. Slide a firm flat surface (thin tray or wooden

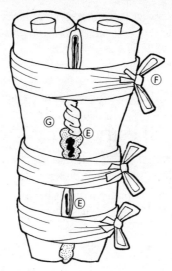

board) under the limb to carry it. Thus swing the limb slowly, carefully, to where you need it.

5. *Protect the Patient against Shock* (see p. 105)

Do not overlook the fact that occasionally a fracture may cause internal, hidden, bleeding which greatly increases the shock risk. A broken rib, for instance, could pierce an organ within the chest or abdomen.

At this point let the student re-read the five steps described above for treatment of fractures and consider how well they exemplify the three basic aims of first aid described on p. xi. These are: 1. to preserve life; 2. to prevent worsening; 3. to relieve pain and discomfort.

Questions

1. Explain the terms 'symptoms' and 'signs' and describe what part they play in your decision as to whether or not an injured person might have broken a bone.

2. Define the 'open' and the 'complicated' fracture. How are they important in the handling of the patient after injury?

3. You find a crowd assembling about a motor-cyclist who has been thrown to the ground after a collision. What are the first two things you should do immediately?

4. What are 'direct' and 'indirect' fractures? Could either of them present a diagnostic problem?

7
Fractures: Specific Sites

You should read this chapter only after having studied the preceding one.

Skull

This is dealt with in the chapter on head injuries (p. 117).

Lower Jaw

In some jaw fractures the patient cannot swallow or spit or is unconscious and he could choke from saliva or blood filling the mouth. Also he could choke from the tongue (which is attached to the jawbone) slipping backwards and blocking the airway at the throat.

1. If necessary clear the mouth very gently: remove any dentures or loose teeth.

2. If he is conscious and his condition is good let him sit up, bending forward to allow fluid to flow out of the mouth.

If he is severly injured or unconscious put him in the Recovery Position (p. 112).

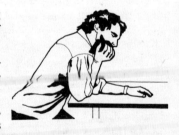

3. Place a thick pad under the jaw, which you support while doing this with the palm of your hand. (If his condition is good the patient can hold it himself.)

4. Now let a wide bandage take the support, passing under the pad, over the ears and knotted at the top of the head. You may use a scarf or a lady's

stocking for this.

5. Watch the patient carefully lest he begins to vomit. Then you would have to remove the bandage and clear his mouth, while supporting the jaw with your hand.

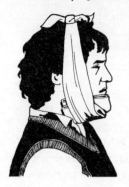

Ribs and Breastbone

When ribs are fractured the pain is aggravated by chest movements; the patient protects himself by taking only shallow breaths. As a rule the muscles which lie between adjacent ribs tend to tense up, acting fairly effectively as natural splints. Therefore it is unnecessary, even inadvisable, to try bandaging across the chest.

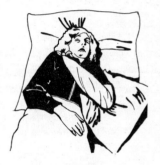

1. Let the patient lie tilted towards the injured side. Place pillows or rolled up material to support his head and shoulders, and also the upper arm and elbow of the injured side.
2. Support the forearm in an elevation sling (p. 19).

Sometimes the pain is only quite slight and the patient is fit enough to sit and walk. However there are rare severe cases of damage to underlying organs with hidden bleeding, or of open wounds into the chest (pp. 36–51). These emergencies need very rapid transport to hospital by ambulance, with the patient lying down, inclined towards the injured side.

Collar Bone

By far the most common causes of this fracture are falls on the side of the shoulder or on the outstretched hand, an example of the indirect fracture (see p. 65). The thin curved collar bone can snap as the result of the transmitted blow.

The features, signs, and symptoms are generally characteristic.

(A) The patient tends to tilt his head towards the injured side as this reduces the painful pull of muscle on the broken bone.

(B) The pain is felt around the shoulder area.

(C) You may be able to see or to feel (very gently!) the irregularity at the break.

(D) The weight of the arm on the injured side aggravates the pain. The patient is likely to be supporting his arm at the elbow.

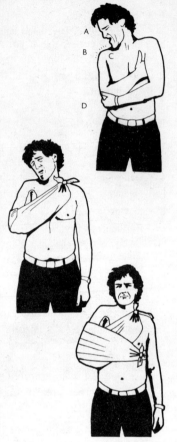

In your treatment make quite sure that this support is maintained until the sling has been properly secured and has taken the weight.

1. On the injured side put padding between the side of the chest and the upper arm and elbow.

2. Gently bring the hand up just below the opposite shoulder.

3. Apply an elevation sling (p. 19).

4. Now further secure the arm to the chest wall by a wide bandage, making the knot on the front of the opposite side.

Remember that, if necessary, the 'elevation sling' could be improvized from a coat jacket (p. 20).

Upper Arm and Forearm

Whenever possible the injured upper limb should be supported in a sling. This means bending the elbow. If, however, the elbow joint area is involved in the fracture it should not be moved. Your treatment there must vary according to circumstances.

If the elbow does not hurt and can be bent

1. Put padding across the chest on the injured side.

2. Gently bend the forearm over the padding, sloping it slightly upwards. Keep it supported.

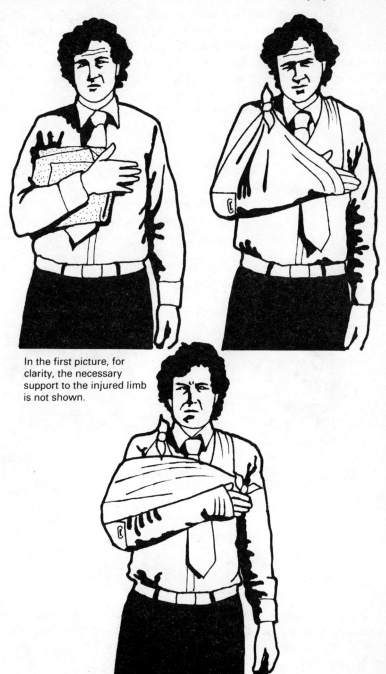

In the first picture, for clarity, the necessary support to the injured limb is not shown.

3. Enclose the elbow and forearm and the padding in an arm sling (p. 18). Remember to let the fingers show beyond the sling and to make the knot in the hollow above the collar bone.

4. Finish with a broad bandage to secure the upper arm to the chest. Make the knot on the front of the chest on the opposite side.

If the elbow hurts but is already bent

Secure the limb as above.

If the elbow hurts, and the limb is straight

Do not try to bend the elbow.

1. Make sure the patient is lying down.

2. Very gently and carefully move the arm alongside his body. He may help himself by using his good hand to keep the arm in position until you have secured it.

3. Place padding between the whole arm and the side of the body.

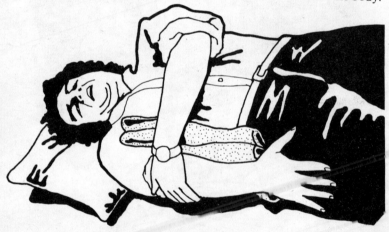

4. Secure the arm to the body by three bandages. You will minimize disturbance if you place them in this order:

    (a) at wrist and thigh level
    (b) at upper arm and chest level
    (c) at forearm and waist level.

Place the knots at the front of the body on the opposite side to the injured arm. Please note that no bandage goes over the elbow itself.

5. Thus strapped the patient cannot walk and will have to be carried by stretcher.

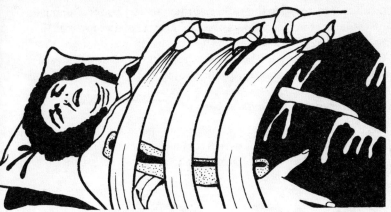

Hand and Fingers

1. Fold generously thick padding over the whole hand.
2. Bend the elbow gently to bring the hand on the chest wall near the opposite armpit.
3. Apply an elevation sling (p. 19).
4. Finish with a broad bandage to secure the whole to the chest wall. Make the knot at the front of the uninjured side.

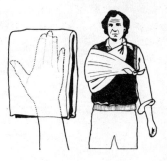

Pelvis

The pelvis is the massive bony ring by which the upper part of the body is supported on the legs. The thigh bones fit into sockets at each side, and the spinal column links into it at the back (see diagram p. 57). Thus a bad fracture of the pelvis would make it difficult or impossible for the patient to walk or stand. Of course a minor fracture of the pelvis might involve only a slight chip of bone at the edge of one of its outer 'wings' and the disability would be much slighter. But to play safe you will treat any suspected pelvis fracture as if it were severe. But you will not need to apply immobilization bandaging unless transport to hospital is likely to prove difficult.

A fracture of the front part of the pelvis might damage the bladder and the urinary tube which leads from it. A consequence of this could be the patient's strong discomfort making him feel that he has to empty his bladder urgently. Were he to do so the urine might escape from the injured parts into surrounding tissues causing even worse troubles. Do not give the patient further anxiety by mentioning this unless he says he needs to pass urine. Then explain only that this is probably due to local irritation from the fracture and that he should try to hold back until he reaches hospital. In hospital he will be safeguarded by the passage of a tube (catheter) to draw away the urine.

When transport to hospital is easy

Keep the patient on his back and let him place his feet in the most comfortable position. If he wishes to bend his knees support them with a pillow or folded coat or blanket underneath. The patient goes to hospital by ambulance.

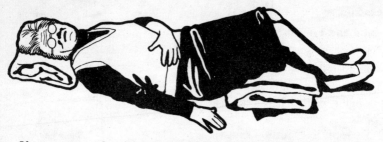

If transport to hospital is difficult or delayed

A wait of half an hour or more, or a journey over rough terrain, needs further precautions.

1. Apply two overlapping broad bandages around the pelvis and hips. Put the lower one on first, and let the second overlap by half the width.

Their purpose is to stabilize and hold in position any disrupted bone. Therefore, although you will be working gently, you must put them on firmly.

Make the knots on the uninjured side (or centrally if you suspect both sides of the pelvis to be fractured)

2. Put padding between the knees and ankles.

3. Tie the feet and ankles together with a figure of eight bandage (p. 22).

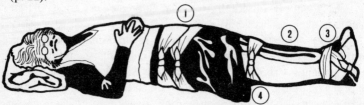

4. Apply a broad bandage firmly round the knees.

Those inexperienced in first aid may make two errors in this treatment. The first is insufficient firmness of bandaging in steps 1 and 4. The second is placing the pelvis bandages either too high or too low, through anatomical uncertainty. You can best learn the position of the pelvis by feeling yourself, rather than by studying a picture. Begin with a hand feeling the hip region. Now by moving the fingers forward and upwards explore and learn the contour of the pelvis bone and its upper and lower limits. This is the area, which should be covered by the bandages.

Fracture in the Leg

The treatment is the same for any part of the thigh and lower leg, with the exception of a fracture in the kneecap, which is described separately.

A common fracture is that of the uppermost end of the thigh bone, especially in elderly people whose bones tend to become brittle. Sometimes only a simple stumble can break the aged bone. Pain is felt about the hip joint.

A characteristic of this fracture is the way the injured leg rotates outwards, so that the foot points sideways. The break has occurred at a level between the attachments of two sets of muscles with opposing actions. One turns the leg inwards; the other turns it outwards. At rest the muscle tone neutralizes each other so that the leg and foot face forward. This balance goes when the fracture separates that action. The thigh bone below the fracture, subjected only to the pull of the one muscle rotates outwards, carrying the leg and foot with it. Remember that this happens only with this particular fracture. The leg may show no rotation if the thigh bone has been broken at another level.

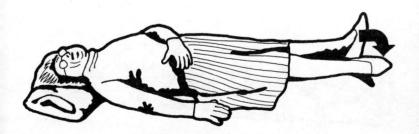

There is another point to remember about fractures near the hip joint. Often the patients (especially the older ones) do not believe that the blow which they have just suffered could have broken a bone, and insist that they merely have a bad sprain. Do not let them dissuade you from being cautious.

When transport to hospital is easy

1. Get the patient lying down. Carefully align the legs together. (If the attempt causes much pain do not try further; maintain the bent position of the broken limb by banking things like cushions or folded blankets around it and await the rescue services.)
2. Put padding between the thighs, knees, and ankles.
3. Tie a figure of eight bandage (p. 22) around the feet and ankles.
4. Bandage the knees together. (However if the fracture seems to be at the knee avoid having a bandage here; put it below this level.)

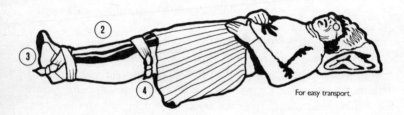

For easy transport.

When transport to hospital is difficult or delayed

You will protect the patient by adding three more bandages.

5. One goes round the lower legs.
6. One goes round the thighs.
7. The last bandage goes below the level of the suspected fracture.

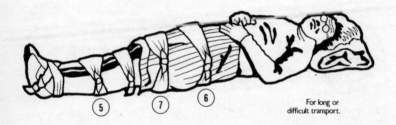

For long or difficult transport.

Kneecap

The kneecap is a small bone in front of the knee joint. It lies within the tough ligament of a large muscle which runs from the thigh to the upper end of the shin bone. It can be broken by a direct blow and also by an abnormally hard action of that muscle (as in trying to right oneself when stumbling or in a hard kick which misses its target).

1. Get the patient lying down. Have his head and shoulders raised on pillows or suitable substitutes.
2. Place a splint like a narrow board under the leg extending from ankle to buttock. Gently raise the leg with the far end of the splint resting on a suitable support.
3. Put padding behind the ankle.
4. Put padding to fill the hollow behind the knee.
5. Secure the ankle to the splint with a figure of eight bandage (p. 22).
6. Bandage the thigh to the splint.

Fix the knots of these bandages on the outer side of the leg and against the splint.

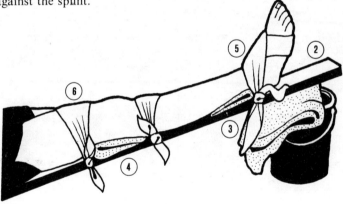

Foot and Ankle

1. Very gently remove the footwear. You do this because the foot may swell so that compression in a shoe or boot threatens its blood circulation. However removing a tall, closely-fitting boot could present such problems of manipulation and pain that you may have to face the choice of leaving it on (if transport to hospital will be rapid) or of carefully cutting and destroying it.
2. Thoroughly encase the foot and ankle within a thick cushion or a

folded blanket; tie on firmly by bandages.

3. Keep the foot elevated as this helps to reduce swelling.

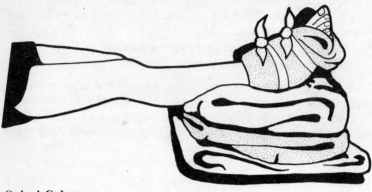

Spinal Column

The spinal column is made up of a number of bones, the *vertebrae* (singular: *vertebra*) sitting upon and jointed to each other. At its summit the column carries the skull. At its base it links with the back of the bony pelvis (diagram on p. 57).

It has two principal functions:

1. Giving stability, with some flexibility to the body's frame.

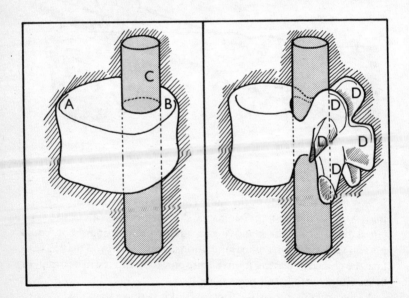

2. Protecting the *spinal cord*, the 'cable' of nerves from the brain carrying sensation and action to and from the brain, serving the various parts of the body.

Although each vertebra has its own characteristics any one can be shown diagrammatically as a fairly thick cylindrical block (A) to which is added, at the back, a bony ring (B). It is through this ring that the spinal cord (C) passes.

The structure of the vertebra is, in fact, much more complicated. The block is irregular in shape and at its sides and rear it has a number of projecting bony processes (D). They help to form the joint between adjacent vertebrae and also are points of attachment for some of the muscles which move the neck and back.

Breaking one or more vertebrae can be a major calamity for the patient. If the fracture involves only a tip of one of the projecting bony processes the matter is not so grave. But if the block or the ring is broken and the pieces of bone shift, then the cord of nerves is in great danger. It may be compressed or even severed. This can cut off power

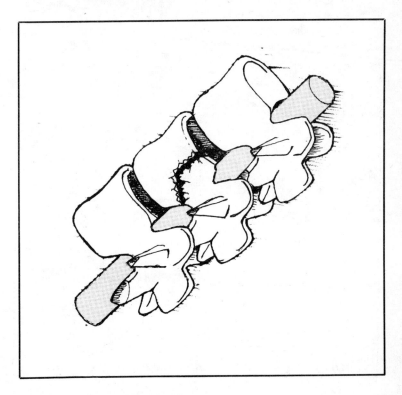

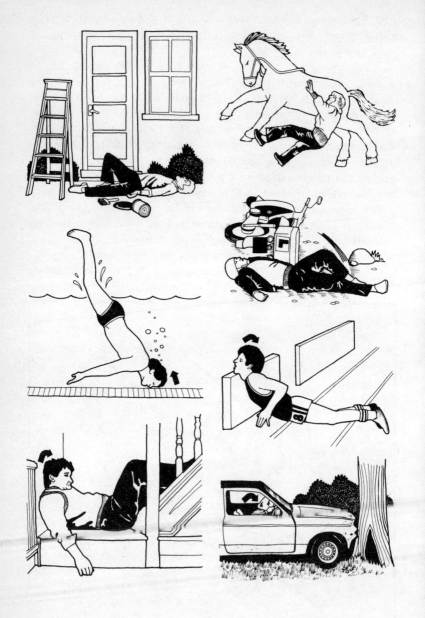

Each of these patients could have a fractured spine.

and sensations to the parts of the body served by the nerves in that region of the cord. In the lower back it could affect the legs; in the neck it could affect arms, trunk, and legs.

Awareness

Always be alert to the possibility of a fractured vertebra. It could happen to someone hit by a heavy object, thrown from a horse, falling from a height, tumbling down a flight of stairs, having head and neck jerked forcibly backwards or forwards in a car collision, landing on his head on diving in shallow water, or even after the impact of coming down on straightened legs after a high jump.

It is a pity that the vertebral column is popularly called the 'backbone'. This does not remind one that the *neck area* should be included. Severe jerking of the head, having it bent suddenly one way or another can fracture a vertebra in the neck.

You must assume a fractured vertebra in all such cases. The accident patient with back or neck pain may have movement and feeling in his hands and feet because the spinal cord has not been damaged ... yet. Broken bone may be waiting to slip against the spinal cord at the first untoward movement of the patient and his vertebral column. The movement may be his because he wants to get up; it may be the helper's because he is ignorant or careless.

When transport to hospital is easy

1. *At once tell the patient to lie still* and prevent bystanders from moving him. Remain by him to ensure this.

2. *Keep his head steady.* The head must not turn or bend sideways. Kneel down and give firm support with one hand on each side of the head. You may be able to delegate a bystander to do this.

3. *Keep the body steady.* You may be able to bank rolled-up coats or blankets or a firm object along each side of the body. Also someone may hold the feet.

4. *Keep the patient warm:* cover him with a blanket or coat.

5. Getting the patient on to a stretcher is a matter for experts (for example, the ambulance attendants). It has to be done so that the patient remains absolutely straight, not only while being lifted but also during transport.

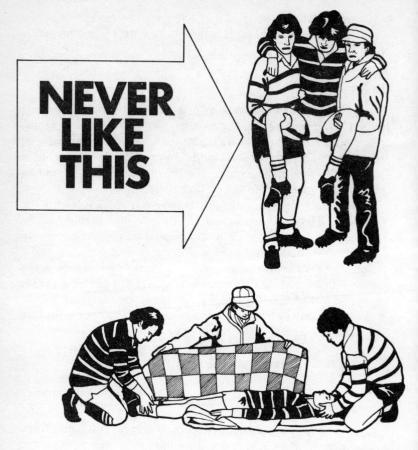

NEVER
LIKE
THIS

The problem is solved by the use of the metal 'scoop stretcher' (also known as the 'orthopaedic stretcher'). After adjusting it to the patient's size the attendants uncouple it at the top and bottom so that it separates down the middle of its length into two pieces. They place each of these halves alongside one or other side of the patient. Then they slide the halves gently towards each other and under the patient without moving him. They couple top and bottom firmly together again. Now they can lift up the patient undisturbed, in the position in which he was found.

When transport to hospital is difficult or delayed

In such cases you must give extra security by extra immobilization. This varies whether the fracture is in the back or the neck.

In the back

Place padding between the thighs and lower legs. Fix the ankles together by a figure of eight bandage. Secure the legs together by two bandages one round the knees and the other round the thighs.

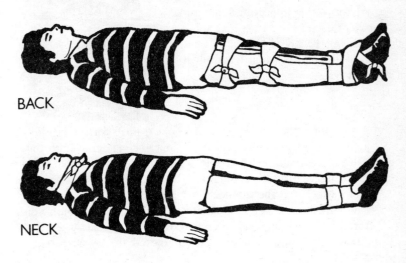

BACK

NECK

In the neck

Ambulance and rescue services carry collar-like splints which are easy to put round the neck. You can improvise something almost as effective. Take a newspaper and fold it so that it is about 10 centimetres wide and 30 centimetres long. (If available newspapers have only a few pages put a couple together.) Slip this inside a woman's stocking or roll a cloth like a triangular bandage (p. 17) round it. This gives two loose ends of material with a firm centre containing the newspapers. Shape this centre into a curve and gently pass the whole behind and round the patient's neck. The newspaper pack fits under his chin and curves closely round each side of the neck. Tie the loose ends of

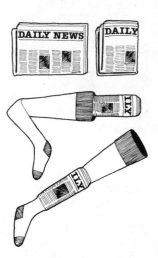

the stocking together at the front. You must do this without moving the patient's neck and head. Have someone supporting the head while you work.

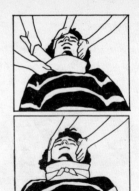

Although the supporting collar is a great protection the fractured spine could still be at risk if the patient moved about. Keep him lying down and at rest.

Dislocations

A dislocation is the displacement of a bone from its correct position at a joint. The circumstances causing it may be very similar to those which cause a fracture. Sometimes a heavy pull can do it; wrenching on the arm, for instance, could get the top of the bone in the upper arm out of its socket at the shoulder.

The patient is in pain and cannot properly move the joint. Some deformity is obvious. Very often it is difficult to decide whether the injury is a fracture or a dislocation. Indeed the two can happen together.

The first-aid answer to this problem is simple. Treat the condition as if it were a fracture, supporting and immobilising the part in the position most comfortable for the patient.

Questions

1. How you immobilise a fractured upper limb depends on whether the elbow seems to be involved. In what way?

2. A man has fallen backwards down a flight of stairs. He ends up with his head bent sharply forwards against a wall. Detail the way you cope. (Ambulance is within easy call.)

3. What risks might threaten a patient who has just sustained a fractured lower jaw and how can you deal with this?

4. Someone is lying on the ground after he has been hit by a car, very hard, in the hip region. How do you help and protect him? (There will be delay in getting an ambulance.)

5. A man in swimming trunks has fractured his collar bone. From the far end of the beach a sharp-sighted, first aider has already made a tentative diagnosis. How?

8
Burns

We tend to think of open flames in connection with burning. Other ways of being burnt are equally powerful and unpleasant: contact with a hot metal; boiling liquids or vapours (scalds); harsh frictional rubbing as on the hands after unskilled sliding down a rope; heat on contact with a live electrical conductor; the corrosive effects of some strong chemicals. All these are forms of burns which cause more or less the same sort of injury. Electrical burn however adds its own type of destruction as well (see pp. 127–8).

Also we tend to think of burns in terms of the harm they do to the surface of the body. This harm is very real, but we must understand how it is related to the heat created, *and retained* in the tissues deep in the skin. The heat is active not only at the moment of the accident; it continues within for quite a long time afterwards. One of its effects is on the blood vessels. These dilate, and are engorged with blood; skin in the burnt area becomes red and puffy.

The blood vessels also become relatively 'porous', letting some of the colourless fluid, part of the blood, ooze out (leaving behind the blood cells). Not only does this increase the general puffiness of the area, but also it collects under and presses up the surface of the skin, forming the characteristic burn blisters. A really extensive area of burn means a large loss of fluid out of the vessels, and no longer in circulation. What is coming out may not look like blood since it is free of the millions of red cells which give blood its colour. But such a drop in the patient's blood volume is quite capable of causing shock (see p. 102) which is life threatening.

Sometimes the skin of the affected area has been burnt away: there is then nothing left to form the roof of the blister. Instead there is a raw open, wet-looking area, from which a lot of fluid may be seeping out. It is not only fluid volume which is being lost to the patient. The fluid is rich in minerals and in proteins—chemicals of importance to the nutrition and well-being of the body. Within its blister covering the fluid remains sterile. However on the surface of an open wound it is exposed to bacteria and infection becomes very likely.

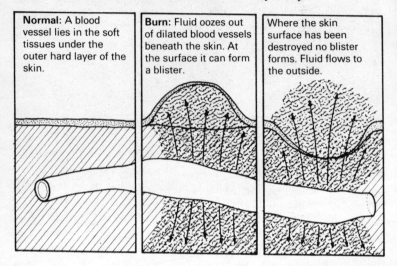

Normal: A blood vessel lies in the soft tissues under the outer hard layer of the skin.

Burn: Fluid oozes out of dilated blood vessels beneath the skin. At the surface it can form a blister.

Where the skin surface has been destroyed no blister forms. Fluid flows to the outside.

Three Basics for Burns

From the above it is clear that first aid to burns involves three basic principles.

1. Give rapid cooling to counter the retained heat in the tissues.
2. Protect the patient against shock.
3. Protect the wound against infection.

Remember that the depth of the wound is of less immediate importance than its area. Obviously, the deeper a burn goes beneath the skin the more it is likely to harm important structures like tendons, nerves or major blood vessels; healing will be less easy and the eventual scar will be worse. But a more superficial burn of far wider extent means a greater zone for plasma loss. Severe plasma loss brings shock (pp. 100–2) and is a threat to life.

Rescue from a Burning Room

Bear in mind that most deaths in buildings on fire are due to choking from heavy fumes. These fumes tend to rise so that the area near the floor is relatively clear.

Have a rope firmly around you, held by someone outside so that he can pull you out should you collapse. Get a wet cloth around your nose and mouth. Breathe in and out twice before you venture in and then

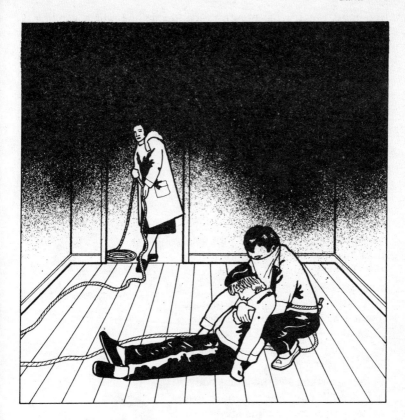

hold your breath as long as you can. Keep low, on your hands and knees if possible. If the fire has been severe, with the chance of the ceiling falling, which is more likely to happen centrally, reach the victim by skirting round the edges of the room. If the victim is unconscious drag him out with your arms under his armpits, and your hands grasped together on the front of his chest. You may find, once you have got him in the open, that he has ceased breathing and needs resuscitation (p. 130).

Warning

Burning of some household furnishings can produce dangerous chemicals in the smoke. They can damage the breathing passages and also act as general poisons. A wet cloth over the face will give no protection; the fire brigade uses special breathing apparatus. If a victim who is rescued from these chemicals needs artificial ventilation you must **not** try the mouth-to-mouth method which would risk poisoning yourself; use the Holger-Nielsen method (p. 145) until specialist help arrives to give oxygen.

Hot Fluids Spilt on Clothing

Get the clothing off at once. The material holds heat and will continue to scald the patient if it is left on. If it is not easy to draw the clothes off, do not hesitate: cut them away.

Clothing on Fire

Extinguish the flames at once. If a large supply of water is handy use this. Otherwise stifle the flames by excluding air from them with any thick material immediately available: rug, blanket, curtain or even your coat.

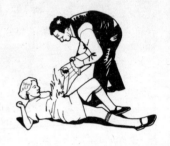

A patient in a panic may be running about which worsens the emergency by fanning the flames. You will have to get him on the ground with the burning part uppermost so that the flames are rising away from his body.

If possible direct the material down on to the patient towards his feet, so that the last of the flames are not fanned on to his head. Press the material firmly against the burning part so as to exclude air and so extinguish the flames.

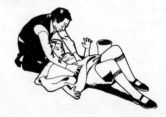

Sometimes one hears advice about rolling the person, who is on fire, on the ground. A little thought shows how unwise this could be. It is difficult to do, and, if achieved, it would mean that different surfaces of the body had been exposed to the flames before they were extinguished. The only possible occasion for rolling would be to do this yourself if you were on fire, with no one present to help and no material to wrap tightly round your body.

After the flames are extinguished

Carefully pull away any charred and *loose* bits of clothing, which may still be smouldering. But do not try to remove more than this, for some cloth may be adherent to the underlying skin, which would come away with it.

Cooling a Burnt Area

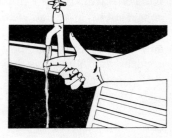

Do this as quickly as you can by using ordinary cold water. (Tests have shown that ice or iced water gives less satisfactory results.)

A finger tip can be held under running water from a tap (but do not allow the water stream to be forceful). A hand or arm can be plunged into a basin or bucket of cold water.

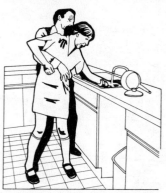

For other body areas, where immersion in water is not practicable, fold a thick cloth like a towel and soak it in cold water. Place it on the burn so that it covers it fully. Apart from its protective action cooling is very effective in reducing pain. Keep it going for *at least* ten minutes. If, at the end of ten or fifteen minutes, the patient still has considerable pain continue the cooling for another ten minutes.

During this time any wet cloth put on may well warm up and start drying. You will then quickly give it a fresh soak in cold water and apply it again.

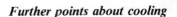

Further points about cooling

Do not be tempted to put the patient into a cold bath. This might seem a logical move with, for instance, a child burnt over a large part of the body. But the effect would be too severe. It is better to use cold wet packs confined to the burnt area. On the other hand it is almost useless to pour water from a jug on to a severe burn. It will run off too quickly. The correct treatment is for the burnt part to have full sustained immersion in, or contact with, the water.

Heat remains quite a long time in the deeper tissues after a severe burn. Even if you arrive on the scene up to half an hour after the accident you should give the cooling treatment.

If a patient with a severe burn is likely to get to hospital by ambulance or to be seen by a doctor within an hour after the accident it would be reasonable to continue the cooling by a wet pack over the burn until the experts take over. Otherwise you will dress it as described below.

The Risks of Swelling

A severe burn causes a lot of swelling. Remove anything which could be caught up within the puffiness and which could constrict. For instance you would take a bracelet or watch strap off the wrist or a ring from the finger before the swelling becomes severe.

You may reduce the extent of swelling in a limb by elevating it. Keep a leg or arm well raised on anything suitable like pillows or folded blankets.

Dressing the Burnt Area

Once you have decided that cooling treatment is complete, you will dress the burnt area like any wound (p. 2). Use sterile dressings or the cleanest material you have. Do not bandage too tightly: let bandaging be just enough to keep the dressing in place.

If no other dressing is available for a burnt arm or leg use a clean pillowcase, as if it were a bag, slip it over the limb and bandage it shut at the top. If you have to cover a burnt face cut some holes in your dressing for the mouth and nose areas so that the patient's breathing is unimpeded.

Do not be misled and apply sprays, lotions or ointments. They have no part in first aid.

The Danger of Shock

This is important. With the severe burn's loss of plasma from the circulation, shock (p. 100) is a real risk and you will take measures against this (p. 105).

Here the general rule against giving anything by mouth should be broken. While you are waiting for a doctor or ambulance and as long as the patient is conscious and co-operative give him half a small cupful of water every ten or fifteen minutes.

Friction Burns and Dry Heat

Flames or hot liquids are not always involved. The touch of very hot metal, for instance, can be just as damaging. Sudden harsh rubbing, for instance contact with the edge of a revolving wheel or movement against a rough cord, can cause enough heat to burn. Treat these with cooling and dry dressing as you would any other burn.

Electric Burns

These are dealt with on pp. 127–8.

Blisters

After the cooling treatment do not disturb any blisters which have formed; carefully include them under the dressing. Opening blisters increases the risk of infection.

Sometimes circumstances will allow you to break this rule. For instance, the heel blistered by a badly-fitting shoe or the blister on an otherwise quite mild burn of a finger tip become mechanical nuisances rather than severe injuries. If medical or nursing aid is not available, then you could justifiably puncture the blister yourself.

Boil a long needle in water for ten minutes. Pour away the water and leave the needle to cool, in its container. Clean the blister and the skin around it with soap and water or a suitable antiseptic (p. 1). Wash your hands. Holding the needle by its blunt end pierce the blister at its base near the skin at a couple of diametrically opposite points. Make the holes large enough to let the fluid pass through easily. Squeeze the fluid out through these holes by pressing down with a sterile or clean cloth. Then put on a clean dry dressing.

This is not likely to work on a blister which is several days old, as the fluid inside will have thickened into a jelly-like consistency.

Chemical Burns

Splashing from harsh and corrosive liquids like strong acids, bleaches or caustic soda also need immediate help with water. In these cases it must be running water, to wash away the chemical. Also quickly remove any contaminated clothes that are holding the chemical.

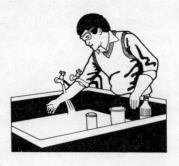

Pour or flow the water copiously until there is no likelihood of any of the chemical remaining, but do not use powerful jets or strong cascades from a high level for they could hurt the burnt area.

Chemicals in the eye

These have their special problems. The patient, in pain, is very likely holding his eye tight shut. You will have to draw his lids apart very gently. Make him lie down towards the injured side, so that the flow of water does not carry the chemical away with it towards the unaffected side. Make sure that your water stream is both generous and gentle.

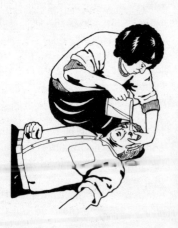

Cover the eye lightly with a dry dressing and get medical help.

Should the patient be wearing a contact lens, you must get it out as soon as possible after starting the wash-out. If it stays in position, it could retain a small amount of the damaging chemical against the eye-ball.

If the patient himself cannot get the lens out try to do it for him. With a finger tip gently pull sideways (away from the eye) the outer junction of upper and lower lids. This draws the lids together; a lid edge will slide against and detach the lens. The patient should be leaning forwards, with the palm of his hand ready to catch the small lens.

Burns in the Mouth

A bad burn in the mouth, whether it be from steam, hot liquids or chemicals is also treated by copious, repeated rinsing out with cold water.

After this you let the patient suck ice-cubes, if they are available. Use of ice is permissible here for the soft tissues lining the mouth may swell very fast and extensively. This could worsen the situation by blocking the airway at the back of the throat. Seek medical help or an ambulance urgently.

Sunburn

Sunburn should not happen to the sensible sunbather who knows that unusual exposure of the skin to sunshine should be gradual, starting with only small areas and for short times.

Get a sunburnt patient into a cool and shady place. Give immediate relief by dabbing the skin gently with cold water and let the patient take pain-easing tablets like aspirin or paracetamol. Also advise him to drink water or fruit juice copiously but slowly.

A helpful application is calamine lotion; the oily form is a little more soothing but can be messy to clothes. Do not let the patient out into the sun again without some light clothing over the sore areas.

If burning is severe, and especially if there are blisters, he should consult a doctor.

Questions

1. Your neighbour calls you to her kitchen where her five-year-old girl is running, screaming, with the front of her dress on fire. Describe in detail all the steps you take.

2. Horses have been driven out of a blazing stable, which is now full of smoke. The stableman however has not emerged. How do you act?

3. In the school laboratory a sixteen-year-old girl has been splashed on a forearm and over one side of her face by strong acid. What do you do?

4. Which is the worse emergency situation; a very deep burn on a small area of the thigh, or a superficial burn with much blistering covering the back? Give your reasons.

9
Shock

The word 'shock' plays a big part in first-aid topics. It is unfortunate that, in the English language it has several meanings and that many of them can be misleading in this context.

'Shock' can stand for a blow. It can cover the effect of electricity on someone. Very often it indicates an emotional reaction – fear or anxiety. None of these covers what is meant when the term is used purely medically.

Shock here means the *physical* way certain injuries and conditions reduce the body's ability to remain alive. It is closely related to inadequate blood supply to tissues because the heart and circulation are functioning badly.

Bleeding and Shock

The clearest illustration of this is the result of severe bleeding after an injury. Imagine an adult man of average size who has just sustained a deep cut to his arm; blood flows freely; before this has been controlled the victim may have lost some three or four pints (about two litres) of blood.

There is significantly less blood going round his body. This will affect the power of his heart since one of the factors that stimulates the heart is the actual volume which enters its chambers between each beat. The heart now acts more feebly. It will beat faster in the attempt to overcome the handicap. Blood is now being pumped relatively inefficiently so that oxygen and nutritional supplies to tissues all over the body are reduced.

Many tissues can manage for a while on these limits. But the brain is extremely sensitive to such deprivation. The victim begins to feel faint. Much more important is the effect on certain important nerve centres in the brain. These govern the working of many factors which keep the man alive. Temperature, blood pressure, respiration and heart action are under their control, which now is becoming poor. In particular the heart beat will be further weakened. A vicious circle is setting in, threatening that man's life force.

This is shock. In the case of bleeding *one can define shock as a progressive failure of the heart and circulation (and of nourishment to body tissues) due to severe blood loss.*

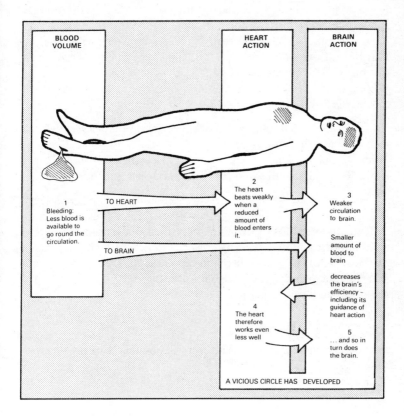

Other Causes of Shock

Many other injuries can have the same effect.

Large bruises

When a bruise is formed the blood remains within the body. It has escaped from damaged blood vessels to pool under the skin (see p. 6) and is no longer playing any part in the circulation.

Large wounds

They may show little blood externally yet may be accompanied by quite a lot of deep bleeding below the skin and within body spaces.

Large fractures

In common with large wounds, large fractures may do just the same. It is not possible to break a bone without, at the same time, damaging organs like the muscles and their blood vessels which lie around or near them. Even if the skin has not been broken, blood will have been lost out of the circulatory system.

Severe burns

These are also potent causes of shock. They bring about a very definite loss of blood fluid (plasma), which oozes out of the heated vessels. Blister formation is an example of this fluid loss on the surface. Deeper down the fluid also fills and swells up the burnt part (see p. 91).

Some medical conditions

A few rare infections of the alimentary tract can cause much loss of fluid into the abdominal cavity. Also a bad heart attack will weaken the working of the heart muscle; in this particular case shock will not be related to loss of blood fluid, but will be directly due to the failing of the circulation's directing pump.

The Picture of Shock

If you examine a shocked patient you will find that there are six signs.

1. *He is pale*

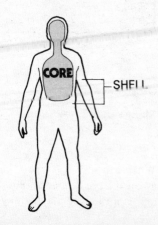

He may show, as well, a blue tinge about the lips, and at tips of nose and ear lobes. The pallor is due not only to impoverished blood circulation but also to a narrowing of the skin's blood vessels. This narrowing is a reflex protective reaction which takes place in arteries serving organs (like the skin) which can make do with less blood during the emergency. As all the arteries under the skin contract they drive out of themselves a great volume of blood. This now becomes available as an extra supply to vessels serving major organs like brain, lungs, and heart muscle—organs that are striving to keep the patient alive. In this situation we can imagine the body as having an outer 'shell' encasing the inner 'core'. The 'shell' is cold and with a minimal blood supply, to allow the 'core' with its life-sustaining organs (brain, heart, lungs, liver) to receive the major share of the available blood, with its warmth.

2. *His skin is cold*

When you touch him he feels cold, as you would expect of a skin which is receiving a markedly decreased blood supply.

3. *He is sweating*

The skin is covered with thin dew-like drops of moisture. The patient feels clammy to the touch.

4. *He is mentally affected*

He may pass from anxiety and restlessness into drowsiness and he may finally become unconscious.

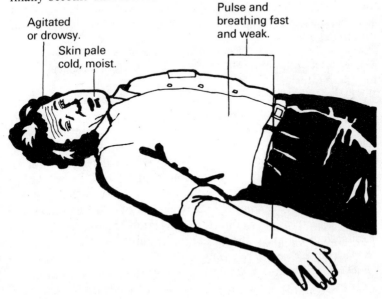

Agitated or drowsy.

Skin pale cold, moist.

Pulse and breathing fast and weak.

5. *His pulse is fast and weak*

Feeling the pulse is described on p. 25. Always do this gently, disturbing the patient and his coverings as little as possible. For instance, you will slip your hand under a blanket rather than pull the blanket back to reach the patient's wrist.

The normal rate of the resting adult's heart beat is 60 to 80 per minute. In shock it may rise to 100 to 150 per minute. The pulse becomes feebler, more difficult to feel, reflecting the weaker action of the heart.

6. *His breathing becomes fast and weak*

The breathing mechanism is considered on p. 37. The adult breathing rate at rest is normally about 16. In shock it can rise to 30 or beyond, with only slight expulsions of the chest wall. In the severest forms of shock, breathing can become a rapid, shallow panting.

As you watch the rise and fall of the chest wall or of clothes covering it, the patient may move or turn, making your observations difficult. But if you began by feeling the pulse do not let go of the wrist as you change to count the breathing rate. Keep your fingers lightly in position. Thinking you are still taking his pulse the patient will not wriggle and will lie co-operatively quiet.

The Development of Shock

The shocked man, described above, is in a bad way. At this point first aid can offer only minor help. He needs all that a hospital can give him, including transfusions.

The thing to learn is that the vicious circle of shock takes time to develop. After the accident the patient's condition gradually sinks towards full shock; it may take minutes or hours according to the severity of the injury or the speed with which blood was lost.

This time allows you the chance to help and to halt the decline of the body's powers. The earlier you attend to this the better will be the patient's chances.

Immediately after some accidents, patients, although emotionally upset, may appear physically fit, and feel it too. Time may prove them wrong; some minutes or hours later the features of shock may begin to show. Your task is *not to treat shock* but, if at all possible, *to prevent shock* or, at least, *to delay and minimise the development of shock*. This means putting into action, as soon as you can, the treatment described below.

If at the very beginning the patient feels in good shape and is unwilling to follow your advice and to get himself looked after properly, you will have to show both understanding and firmness. Give not so much advice as instructions, making it clear that as first aider you are in charge and that you know what is needed. Do not wait for him to worsen.

Anti-shock Measures

1. *Stop bleeding at once* (see p. 27)

This, of course, takes priority, unless the patient has the additional complication of not being able to breathe, which also must be seen to at once (p. 39).

2. *Position and rest the patient*

(a) Move him as little as possible. Treat him where he is.

In settings of immediate danger to both of you, for instance, a house on fire, a gas-filled room or a building liable to collapse, you would have to break this rule. In a road accident, until the police come, use bystanders to direct cars clear from the scene.

(b) Lie the patient down, preferably in the Recovery Position to safeguard his breathing (see p. 112).

(c) If possible keep his head low and his legs raised; this helps circulation towards the chest and brain. You can raise the foot end of a stretcher or bed some 45 to 60 cm. (1½ to 2 feet) by a chair or suitable prop underneath. A patient on the ground can have his legs raised on sacks, rugs or boxes.

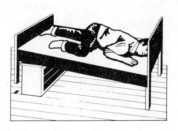

All handling must be gentle. However beware of moving a patient who may have a fracture, especially if his back or neck is involved. In some cases it will be best to keep him in the position in which you have found him.

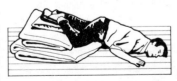

3. *Prevent heat loss*

Ensure this by covering him with a rug, blanket, coat or sacking. This

should be comfortably loose and not
fitted tightly. Unless he is on suitably
heat-insulating material, like a mattress or a thick carpet, try to get him
protected underneath as well.

But you must **not** add extra heat
like hot-water bottles or an electric
blanket. You should be protecting the
patient against getting colder, but you
should **not** aim to warm him up. Were
you to do so the extra heat would
dilate his skin vessels; they then would
take in more blood. His skin might
become pink again but that would
show how the 'shell' of the body has
drawn blood away from the 'core',
depriving vital organs of some of the
blood they need in the present emergency.

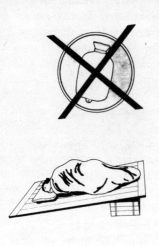

4. *Relieve pain and discomfort*

Pain and mental anxiety do not by themselves cause shock, but they
can aggravate it. Do all you can to ease the patient. You should not
give any tablets or medicine unless told to by a doctor. Much pain can
be relieved by efficiently dressing wounds and by immobilising
fractures. You will also allow the patient to adopt his position of
greatest comfort provided this does not interfere with your care to his
injuries, and to possible fractures or with your protection of his
breathing (see p. 52).

Loosen any constricting clothing such as belts, braces, collars,
disturbing him as little as possible.

Your demeanour will play a very powerful role in reassuring him.
Even if you feel very concerned about the patient's safety (or about
your own expertise) show a methodical and outwardly confident
manner. Begin by explaining that as a first aider you can help him. Do
not work in silence but talk to him quietly, sympathetically, and also
firmly. Explain simply without fuss what you are doing and why,
always stressing how you are getting things under control.

Answer any questions as accurately as you can, dwelling on
comforting and positive aspects only. Never put the patient off with
disquietingly vague platitudes like 'Don't worry'.

Tactfully but very firmly clear away any agitated or demoralising bystanders. If necessary get them off the scene by giving them things to do—such as boiling some water or seeking some equipment which, in fact, you may not necessarily need.

Never whisper to others near the patient, who would immediately assume the worst. Nor be misled by a patient's appearance of unconsciousness. He may yet be able to hear and register mentally what is said near him. By his side restrict your statements only to those things which would help him psychologically if he heard them (see also p. 224).

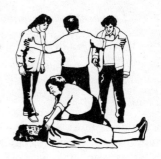

5. *Give nothing by mouth*

Do not give hot tea or coffee or any other food or drink. After a bad injury the patient could vomit. Anything he brings up might then be aspirated into his windpipe and choke him, especially if he is comatose or is later given an anaesthetic for emergency surgery.

If he is very thirsty wet his lips or let him suck a moist cloth: this can be effective in refreshing him without any significant amount of water being swallowed.

Brandy and whisky are false stimulants and you must not allow them to be given. They can dilate the blood vessels in the patient's skin, with the same bad effect as would come from warming him.

Also it is unwise to let the patient smoke. In his condition even one cigarette could be detrimental by decreasing the activity of the heart

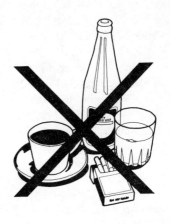

and reducing the oxygen-carrying capacity of the blood.

6. *Get medical help or ambulance quickly*

See pp. 216, 225 about sending messages for help.

Fainting

Fainting is unlike shock. It is due to a temporarily inadequate blood supply to the brain. An emotional upset (fright, displeasing sight, bad news) can cause this. So can pain, fatigue, standing for long periods or a hot, stuffy atmosphere.

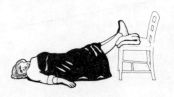

Before becoming unconscious the patient feels giddy and unsteady. He becomes pale, with a feeling of coldness and clammy sweat. His pulse is weak but (unlike the pulse in shock) it is slow. His vision may blur.

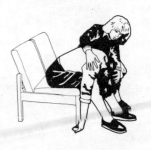

At this stage you help him by getting him to lie down, and by raising his legs above the level of his chest. If circumstances prevent lying down, as when he is seated in a crowded hall, let him bend forwards as far as he can, with his head well-down, between his knees.

Loose any tight clothing at the neck, chest and waist. Ask him to breathe slowly and deeply. Open the window for fresh air.

As soon as he has improved sufficiently to manage it, let him sip cold water. Keep him lying a few minutes after he seems to have recovered; most of those who have felt faint try to get up too soon.

Sometimes fainting is more likely after having missed a meal. Once he has recovered ask the patient about this and, if necessary, advise him to take sweetened drinks.

If the patient has fully fainted or is drowsy, treat him as for unconsciousness (p. 110). Do not try to make him drink, for in this state he could choke.

Questions

1. Briefly outline the six basic first-aid measures of combating the development of shock.

2. An elderly man in the cinema seat next to you suddenly feels faint. How do you help him?

3. Describe all your measures to reassure a badly injured patient while you treat him.

4. What are the likely findings as you examine a patient who is developing shock?

5. List the types of injury which can cause shock. What is the common factor to them all?

10
The Unconscious Person

How should you act if you discover someone who is unconscious? You have spoken to him, you have touched him and he shows no response. What are the next steps?

There are many who, erroneously, would now try to lift or turn him. Others may leave him and hurry off to get help. They too would be mistaken, however good their intentions.

It is natural to query what it was that made the person unconscious, to hunt around for a reason. Unless the cause is life threatening and immediately correctable, such as asphyxia (p. 39) or severe bleeding (p. 27), this is only a secondary factor in first aid. It certainly is a major diagnostic matter for the doctor who will see the patient. But the first aider should learn that, whatever brought it about, it is the unconsciousness itself which can threaten the patient's safety by threatening his airway.

You need a planned approach.

1. Has the patient stopped breathing?

Bend low over him: look and listen. If he is not breathing you begin resuscitation at once (p. 130).

2. Can he breathe properly?

He may be making respiratory efforts but not managing to get air easily in and out of his chest. Either there is silence or from the throat there may be harsh rough sounds of air trying to overcome an obstruction.

The obstruction could well be the patient's own tongue which has flopped against the back of the throat. This is particularly likely to happen if the patient is lying on his back with his head bent forward (p. 49).

Fully, but gently, bend his head backwards which lifts the tongue and clears it from the throat. Do this without turning the head sideways, for that could worsen any fracture sustained at the neck. Once the airway is clear the patient may now gasp in a deep breath, fill his lungs and then be able to breathe in and out normally.

If he is still not breathing easily he may be choking from something else like food, displaced dentures or blood blocking the airway. Immediately look in the mouth. You will use your curved forefinger to scoop out anything from it (see p. 41). If necessary follow up with the routine for treating choking (see p. 42).

In any case always look in the mouth in case there is something there to be removed before it gives trouble.

3. Look for wounds and bleeding

You must control severe bleeding at once (p. 27). Sometimes when breathing has been poor or absent, a wound will not bleed much. As soon as you have restored effective breathing the patient's heart beat and circulation improve, blood flow strengthens and the bleeding shows up. Look over all the patient for signs of blood or of dampness and staining on clothing.

If you find open wounds, which are not bleeding, cover them with any dressing you have with you or can improvise (see p. 2).

Do all this with the minimal disturbance of the patient's position. If possible do not move him at all until you have completed the next step.

4. Try to judge if there are any fractures

A limb bent in an abnormal way is obvious. But this happens to only a minority of fractures. The other diagnostic signs of swelling or localised deformity (p. 68) may not be easy to find. Try by systematic feeling. Do not prod with your finger tips. Feel with the flat of both hands, one on each side of the part you are palpating. This way you are not likely to move any broken bone.

Start at the top of the head, and work slowly downwards. Then feel the shoulder and collar-bone areas. Now move down each arm to the hand. Feel all round the pelvis and then move down each leg. If you discover a knobliness which puzzles you check whether it is present on the other side of the body, in which case it is not likely to be a fracture but a

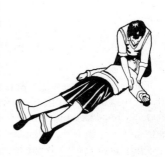

normal anatomical structure.

It can be very difficult to diagnose a fractured spine in someone who is unconscious. Try by sliding your hand under his neck and then under his back, carefully feeling for an irregularity. All too often such palpation is unlikely to give enough information. The golden rule is that *if circumstances suggest there might be a fractured spinal column, then it is fractured* until expert examination and, perhaps, X-rays prove otherwise (see p. 69). For instance, if the patient has fallen from a height, been thrown from a motor-cycle, or received a blow to his head then you must assume that he could have broken his spinal column. You must not move him. Keep this in mind in accidents to football or rugby players, to swimming-pool divers and to horse riders.

Should you find what you suspect to be a fracture you now have to work out how best to immobilise it (p. 71) before you move the patient. Indeed in some cases it may be wise not to put him in the Recovery Position described in the next step, but to leave him in his present position and to make sure that his head remains fully bent back so that he can breathe.

5. *Put the patient in the recovery position*

Unless you suspect a fracture, which you cannot immobilise, you move him into this position, which ensures his stability and protects him from choking. He is lying on his side with:

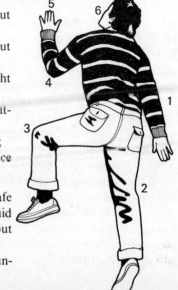

1. the lower arm stretched out straight behind the body;
2. the lower leg stretched out straight;
3. the upper leg bent at a right angle at the hip and at the knee;
4. the upper arm bent at a right-angle at the elbow;
5. the upper hand near the face;
6. the head tilted back and the face bent down.

This position keeps the patient safe with the airway clear. Any fluid (saliva, blood, vomit) will flow out and not run into his windpipe.

The technique to move an unconscious person into this position is simple.

Begin by emptying his pockets of anything that could be uncomfortable to lie on. Remove spectacles he may be wearing. Loosen tight clothing at the neck or waist. Kneel down near his side and cross his further foot over the nearer ankle. Move his further forearm to lie across the chest. Line his nearer arm alongside the body, tucking it well into the side. Turn his head towards you and tilt it back. He is now ready to be turned on to his side.

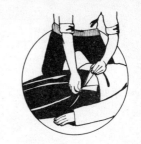

Grasp his further hip firmly and roll him over towards you, against your knees and thighs. At the same time use your other hand to cradle his head and support it, so that it does not bump on the ground as it comes round.

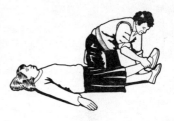

Adjust the head and limbs into their correct positions before you leave your kneeling position which is supporting the patient. If he is lying in rough or muddy soil you could lay a flat cloth under his head. But you should never raise the head on a pillow.

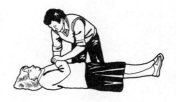

Even a large, heavy patient can be moved this way with someone's help. Your assistant can look after the head while you grasp and turn with one hand on the hip and the other on the shoulder. Or the assistant could push from the other side as you do the turning.

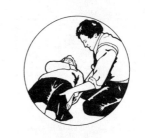

Use the Recovery Position also for weak, injured or drowsy patients who may vomit or may be likely to lapse into unconsciousness.

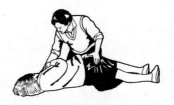

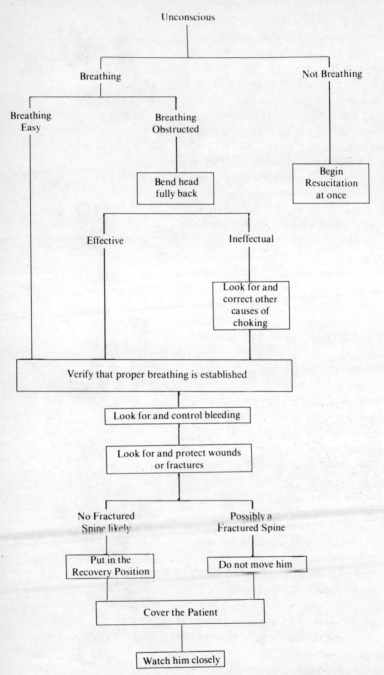

6. Cover the patient

This may mean covering him loosely with a blanket or coat.

7. Keep watching him

While you await help, keep watching your patient. He may vomit and need his mouth clearing out. He may even stop breathing and need resuscitation.

Of course you must never try to give anything to drink to the unconscious or drowsy person. He cannot swallow and the fluid could choke him.

You may find a card in the pocket, wallet or handbag or a disc at the wrist with information that the patient suffers from some condition like diabetes or epilepsy. Pass it to the ambulance attendant or doctor.

Perhaps your patient smells strongly of alcohol. Do not dismiss him as 'only drunk'. He may have stumbled and fallen; he may have had a stroke; he may have some severe abdominal reaction to his drinking. He is at as great a risk as any other unconscious person.

An unconscious patient with suspected fractured spine whom you have found and kept lying on his back may suddenly show signs of vomiting. You have the serious problem of trying to turn him on his side before vomit chokes him. This must be done without any bending of his neck or back and, ideally, several helpers are required. One will cradle, steady and gently stretch the patient's head with a hand on each side. Another will hold and gently pull on the legs. One or two will control the trunk and buttocks. When all are ready the order is given and the patient kept straight as he is turned 'in one piece'. Maintain this support and clean his mouth until the vomiting ceases.

The Patient's General State

Unconsciousness is a relative term, for insensibility has various degrees. A patient's lowered level of responsiveness has been classified as follows.

1. He may not talk except to reply only when you question him directly.
2. His answers will be vague and distant.
3. He does not answer, but he will obey those commands you make.
4. There is no response except to pain. He is motionless, but will withdraw a hand when you pinch it.
5. He is quite inert and shows no response to anything.

A patient may move from one level to another before he is attended to by a doctor. Make a careful note of the time you first see the patient and the level at which you found him, and let the doctor know this; the information can prove very valuable.

Other facts you should give the doctor or write down to send with the ambulance are:

what happened to the patient before he lost consciousness; bystanders could tell you;
the colour, dryness, moisture, heat or coldness of the skin;
the pulse and breathing rates;
any special odour of the patient's breath;
if the patient has vomited;
whether the pupils of his eye are abnormally widened or narrowed, or whether they are unequal (see p. 121).

If there is a long wait for the doctor or the ambulance make your observations every fifteen minutes and write them down. The doctor will be greatly helped by these facts.

Fainting

See page 108.

Epilepsy

See page 193.

Questions

1. From consciousness to unconsciousness there are several levels. Describe them.

2. At the foot of scaffolding, by a slipped ladder, you find an unconscious workman. A bystander has run up and is about to turn him into the Recovery Position. What is your role?

3. Describe how the patient lies in the Recovery Position. Explain the reasons for the way (a) the upper leg and arm; and (b) the head are placed.

4. Your grandfather has not come down to breakfast. You find him in bed, propped against pillows, breathing noisily and quite unconscious. What is your first action and why?

5. What circumstances would make you decide not to put an unconscious patient in the Recovery Position?

11
Head and Brain

This chapter begins with a warning. Some obvious head injuries are accompanied by the more hidden, and potentially more dangerous, fractures of the spine, especially in the neck region. You must approach all patients who have received severe blows to the head with this in mind. The important precautions to prevent damaging movement and to stabilise the spinal column are described on p. 87.

Fractured Jawbone

See p. 74.

Fractured Skull

Imagine a hollow sphere which is brittle but nevertheless has a certain elasticity. If it receives a strong blow at its top or side it will tend to flatten from top to bottom and also to spread out sideways. The force of the blow may crack it at the point of impact. On the other hand the compressed sphere could have its greatest disruption about half-way down at its equator.

The upper part of the skull can be considered as an incomplete sphere. Half way down, and inside, is the *base of the skull*, the irregular shelf on which the brain rests. If the head receives a blow a fracture may happen where it is hit (1); this is a direct fracture (see p. 64). But it may instead (or as well) suffer damage at the level of its greatest width, causing a fracture of the base of the skull (as at 2 and 3); this is an indirect fracture.

You must always think of this possibility when dealing with the patient whose head has been hit. In the case of the direct fracture there may be swelling of the scalp and perhaps an open wound.

The indirect fracture in the base of the skull will not show outwardly in the same way. But sometimes it gives a clue which should not be disregarded. Some parts of this bony shelf are very thin and break

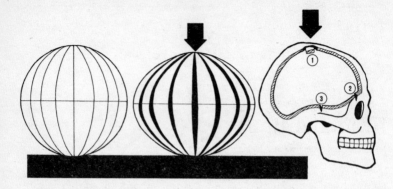

easily, especially in front near the nose and the orbit of the eye and towards the rear by the ear. Fractures at those points could cause bleeding to show from the nose, or around the eye (as a 'black eye' bruise) or from the ear canal.

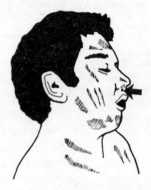

The escaping blood may be quite slight in amount and not dangerous in itself. Sometimes it can appear thin and watery, carrying with it some of the fluid that lies within the membranes which are folded round the brain. In a face, which has received many cuts and abrasions, do not let all the marks and bleeding on the damaged skin make you overlook a small but significant touch of blood from the nostril or from the ear canal. Such a patient urgently needs medical care.

First Aid for a Head Injury

1. Guard the spinal column. Unless the patient is fully conscious and it is clear that there is no pain in the neck and back take the precautions described on p. 87.

2. Guard the patient's airway if he is not fully conscious or is not breathing easily (p. 110).

3. Control any severe bleeding (p. 27).

4. Dress any open wound. After a heavy blow even a small cut of the scalp or forehead could overlie a break of the bone; there is a risk of infection passing beyond this open fracture to the brain beneath it.

5. Place the patient in the Recovery Position (p. 112). If there is blood from the ear canal or from the nostril he should be lying on or towards the side of the bleeding (p. 34).

6. Protect him by covering the trunk and limbs with blankets or coats.

7. Send for an ambulance or doctor.

8. Watch the patient carefully lest he vomit, needs help to his airway or develops abnormal signs.

Brain Damage

A hard blow to the head, whether or not it breaks the bone, may affect the brain itself. It can happen in two different ways, called *concussion* and *compression*.

Concussion

This is the 'knock out' which makes the patient unconscious immediately on receiving the blow. He lies completely unmoving, toneless, pale and with a feeble pulse. Concussion is jarring of the brain. However there is no structural brain damage and in a short time (seconds or minutes) the patient recovers consciousness. Your treatment is, as for all cases of unconsciousness (p. 110), with concern over the possibility of a fractured spine (p. 112). When the patient recovers he may have some irritability and headache. He may even show loss of memory for what happened just before the accident and, literally, not know what hit him.

He must rest and get medical advice. Do not allow him to resume the task or sport in which he had been engaged. Immediate return to activity could considerably worsen and lengthen the headache. Also, more importantly, at this stage you do not know whether he might yet develop compression.

Compression

Increasing pressure may be exerted on the brain. There can be several causes. A piece of fractured bone may be depressed against the nervous tissue. There may be bleeding within the skull. Also the brain may become puffy and swollen as does any other soft part of the body after it has been injured.

Many organs inside the body have greater natural movement and 'give' than is realised by the non-anatomist. If some part swells or is slightly displaced then the adjacent structures generally shift and adapt with little or no decrease of efficiency. Pressure from bruises on to neighbouring tissues give no more than temporary inconvenience. Even the displaced bone of a fracture (unless it is a large or complicated one) is likely to be accommodated by the area concerned.

Such latitude is not for the brain. Here is an extremely sensitive organ, jelly-soft and closely confined by the hard bone of the skull. Any addition within that space can severely upset its function.

Swelling and pressure may gradually increase. The brain is pressed on the inner aspects of the skull. Its lowest part is pushed down to be jammed against the only exit. This is the round, hard-edged aperture of the skull through which the brain stem passes to become the beginning of the spinal cord. It is this brain stem which contains the nerve centres that control functions of life, such as heart beat and respiration.

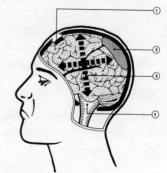

COMPRESSION: CAUSES AND EFFECTS

1. Broken bone
2. Blood clot
3. General swelling.
4. Brain stem in its aperture from the skull.

The dimensions involved are very small but with a sensitive, nerve-packed structure (i.e. the brain) the effects are great.

At first the patient may appear relatively unaffected. As compression proceeds his mind becomes clouded and his life power threatened. Eventually, in hours or even days, he could become confused, comatose, and then unconscious.

There may be other features as compression builds up. Generally the pulse and breathing rates slow down; a worsening headache appears; the patient may vomit; he may become irritable and irrational; he may dislike light and keep his eyes shut. All these are variable and you must not be falsely reassured by their absence.

Coexisting concussion and compression

Very often a head blow gives both conditions. The patient becomes unconscious immediately because he is concussed. After a while he comes out of this and seems to be clear-minded again, or at least partly conscious.

Meantime more serious injury within the skull sets up the beginning of compression. After a characteristic *lucid interval* the patient returns to lowered awareness, perhaps with headache and dizziness, until he becomes drowsy and then unconscious again. The length of the lucid interval can be very variable, ranging from half an hour to a day or more. That is why it is so important to keep a watch on someone who has come to after concussion: at this stage there is no guarantee that compression will not supervene.

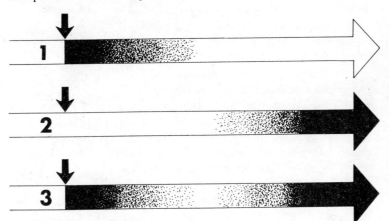

In the diagram time moves from left to right with arrows at the moment of the accident.
A normally conscious patient is shown by white bands; black is total unconsciousness; grey areas are degrees of decreased consciousness in between.
1. Concussion.
2. Compression.
3. Concussion followed by compression with a lucid interval between.

One other possibility is the patient who is knocked out at once by concussion but who remains unconscious with no sign of improvement. In this person compression has occurred as well, so fast that it caused its own unconsciousness before the patient recovered from that due to concussion.

Compression and the Eyes

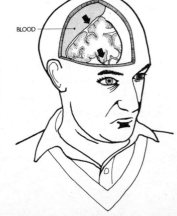

The iris, the coloured ring of the eye, is a muscle which changes size to regulate the amount of light going through the dark, central pupil. The nerve which controls this muscle comes to it from the brain.

Rising pressure on one side of the brain may reach and stimulate the nerve; this in turn activates the muscle of the iris and contracts the pupil on that side.

If your patient with a head injury shows pupils of unequal size, suspect brain compression. Sometimes the comparisons between pupils may alter as the condition worsens.

The patient may begin with both pupils equal and of normal size (1).

Then, for instance, the right pupil may become smaller due to compression acting on that side (2). However any nerve and muscle that is long stimulated and irritated will eventually cease to function. The iris muscle will then totally relax and so the right pupil will become abnormally large (3). Finally compression may extend to affect the nerve and iris of the other side, and the left pupil will contract (4). In fact every combination of size and inequality could show up on examining the eyes.

Do not believe that because the patient shows equal pupils he could not therefore be suffering from brain compression. If a contracted pupil is about to become abnormally wide, it will pass through a stage when it is of normal size. On the other hand, the brain may be suffering a severe degree of compression but not in the area holding the nerves to the iris, so that pupils do not alter.

Finding unequal pupils is of significance. But if your patient has equal pupils it is not necessarily reassuring.

Head Injury and Hospital

Details of the development of compression may seem only of academic interest to the first aider. There is little or nothing specific that he can do about them.

When doctors at hospital receive the patient they can judge what has been happening inside his skull in two ways. The first is by careful clinical examination. Second, and as important, is the story of how and when the accident happened and of the patient's appearance and behaviour after this.

Whenever you send the patient to medical help, try to let the doctor have a written report of:

1. what was the accident;
2. its time;
3. when you first saw the patient and what was his state;

4. what you did in the way of dressings, immobilisation, and so on.

Now, if there is any delay before the ambulance can arrive, and you remain for some time with the patient record carefully every quarter or half an hour your findings on:

1. the patient's degree of consciousness (p. 115);
2. his pulse and breathing rates (pp. 25, 104);
3. his pupils;
4. any special features like headache, nausea, vomiting or twitching of a limb (state which).

Such help can prove of immense value to the doctors and, ultimately, to the patient.

Questions

1. As you and your patient, with a head injury, are high on a mountain it will be several hours before the stretcher party arrives to take him to hospital. Describe the sort of notes you would send with him.
2. The patient, whom you attend after his head injury, has a very small left pupil and the right one is normal in size. He becomes drowsier and then you find that both pupils are of normal and equal size. Is this a disquieting or a comforting point, and why?
3. You run to reach someone who has just been thrown from a motor-cycle on to his head. He is very dazed but just beginning to try to move. What urgent first steps do you take? And what is the rest of the first-aid treatment?
4. What do you understand by 'Brain Compression'? What are the ways this compression could happen?
5. The hero of an adventure story is hit on the head with a bottle and knocked out long enough for the villain to abduct the heroine. As soon as he comes to the hero gives chase in his powerful sports car.

Were you his passenger how would you help and advise him?

12
Electricity

Electric current could in some respects be compared to the current of water coming from a waterfall.

The effect of an encounter with the flowing water depends on the *force* of flow, that is the *height* of the waterfall from which it started.

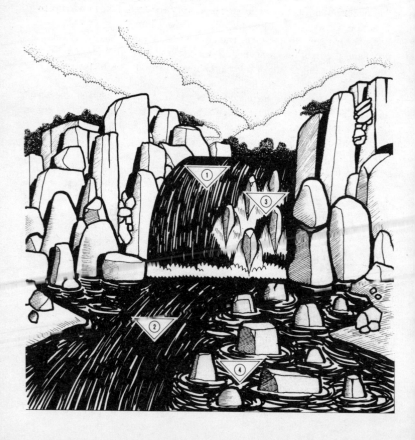

An easy unimpeded fall (1) will give a fast rushing flow in the river (2). However the water's journey may be resisted and broken up on the way by twists and turns or interposed barriers like rock (3); then its rush will be weakened and the flow will be slower (4) or stopped.

The electric current's parallel to the initial force due to the waterfall's height is its *voltage*. *Resistance* to the flow is also a factor. Electricity flows easily and strongly in good conductors like metal and water. But in resistant or insulating materials like wood, rubber or thick cloth it flows weakly or not at all.

Just as the major interest about a waterfall is its height, so one important factor in the way electricity can hurt the body is its voltage. The higher the voltage the greater the immediate threat to life—unless really adequate insulation is interposed.

But even low voltages can prove dangerous. The *type of contact* plays a part. Dry skin is a poor conductor of electricity. Wet skin on the other hand is a good conductor and this includes skin made moist by sweat. Another factor is *earthing*. Electric current selects a path to the earth if there is one available.

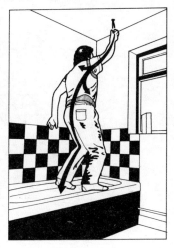

On its way to earth the *current's path through the body* is significant. There may be but a small point of entry where the victim touched a live, electric conductor, but then the current can spread out to many organs. It may pass dangerously through the region of the heart or important nerves of the spinal cord, with very severe results such as stopping of heart beat and breathing. The careless householder in the picture with his hands on a live wire and one wet foot on the bath tub (earthed through its water pipes) is open to just such a calamity.

Effect of Electricity on the Body

It will burn at the point it enters. A small dark skin mark may be the tip of a wide and deep, conical-shaped spread of damage through the tissues beneath. In its path electricity clots blood vessels or ruptures them, causing bruises and areas denuded of blood supply. Brain and other nerve tissue are easily injured; unconsciousness and paralysis could result. If touched by electricity the heart muscle will go into weakened and disorganised rhythm, or even stop beating. On ordinary muscle some electric currents cause unrelaxed spasms of contraction. This could mean that a victim who grasped an unsafe apparatus culd not let go. His fingers would be tightly clenched on to it as long as the current flowed. Finally at its exit point electricity could burn severely. The rash man in the picture above might acquire small superficial burn marks on his fingers and deep ulcerated burns on the sole of the foot which touched the metal bath edge.

First Aid

Do not touch the victim until he is free from the current.

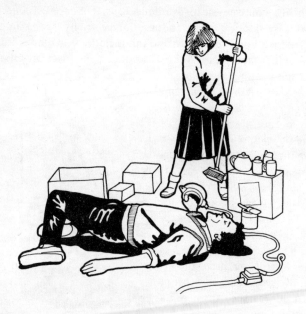

1. *Free the patient from the electricity*

The force of the electric shock may have thrown him clear from the live contact. But if he is still in contact.

  (a) *switch the electricity off.* If this cannot be done

  (b) *pull the connecting plug from the socket.* If this cannot be done

  (c) *disconnect the plug by pulling on the cable.* If this cannot be done

  (d) *push or knock the victim from contact using a non-conductor.*

You can use wood (broom handle, wooden stick, wooden chair). Or get your hands *well inside* thick folds of *dry* material (e.g. a rug or coat) and push with that. You can pull with a loop of rope (or scarf or tights) thrown round the apparatus, or the patient. As a last resort, with thick, dry (and, preferably, rubber-soled) footwear you can kick the victim free as you run past him.

2. Check if he is breathing

You may have to give resuscitation (p. 130).

3. Look for any other injuries

The force of a fall may have caused fractures or wounds which should be protected. In particular look for and dress burns at the exit and entry points of the current. Sometimes the electric burn looks very slight on the skin. But, because of the deep damage they can do, all such burns should have expert opinion.

4. Send the patient to hospital by ambulance

Do this unless the shock has been quite mild with no skin marks or general effects. Keep him under observation for he may show a delayed collapse.

A Car in Contact with Wires

It can happen that electric wires fall over the roof of a motor car. This would make the car electrically alive, but its occupants are safe since the car is not earthed. It is raised off the ground on rubber tyres.

The driver and passengers must try to escape by opening the door and jumping out so that their feet reach the ground only when their hands and the rest of their body are clear of the car and not touching it.

Extremely High Voltages

Ordinary domestic electricity is at 200 to 250 volts. Industry can have far higher values. Factory voltage may rise to 1,000 or more, but is covered by stringent safety regulations.

Extremely high voltages of several hundred thousand volts are found in power stations, in the overhead cables of electric railways and in the pylons of the electricity transport system. They can instantly kill anyone who not only touches but simply gets near to them. The electricity here has the power of sparking out across distances. If you see anyone so hit, *keep away*. An attempt at rescue at this stage would create a second victim—you.

Immediately notify the authorities (police, electricity board) and prevent bystanders from approaching. Stay at least 20 metres (70 feet) from the electric point until the electricity has officially been declared as cut off. Unfortunately the victim's chance of survival will have been extremely small.

The Small Electric Burn

Sometimes a brief touch on a live electric point gives the patient fortunately no more than quite a slight shock and a small dark spot on his skin.

However this visible spot could be the tip of a wide, deeper wedge of damage where the spreading current has burned tissues and closed off their blood vessels. Advise the patient to consult his doctor in case medical supervision is needed.

Lightning

Lightning seeks to be earthed through the easiest route. Its zigzag path shows changes of direction through the most moist and best-conducting bands of air. Approaching earth it will go for sharp prominences or bumps on smooth surfaces. A human being standing free from his surroundings or alongside a high vertical object could be hit by lightning.

Once he has been struck the electricity has come and gone. It is quite safe to handle the patient at once. Your first aid to him is as for other electric attacks. He may have been thrown some distance by the blow, so fractures are likely. Also you may have to cover irregular scorching marks on the skin; forked and zigzag like the lightning itself they show paths of electricity over the victim's trunk.

Safety in Thunderstorms

Avoid being prominent or being near a prominent structure. You are relatively safe within a forest of many trees, but at risk if alongside a single tree in a field. If you must be by a tree keep well away from its trunk: crouch down just beyond the outer edge of the foliage spread.

Crouching in depths and hollows of land and under the protection of an overlying ledge is better than standing free on flatness or at summits. Keep away from small huts, pylons, towers, tents, metal fencing, metal clothes-lines, and bicycles. Do not hold umbrellas. A group of people should spread out so as to have several yards between each person.

The safest place is indoors (away from chimneys, fireplaces and windows). A metal or metal-roofed building will be good shelter (provided you do not touch the metal), and so will a metal-roofed car. A tent gives no protection; a metal pole and wet canvas can be dangerous.

Anyone in water or on a boat should make for the shore.

Questions

1. In a field near the farm a man has been electrocuted by the fall of a high power cable across his tractor (which is now stationary). What should be done?

2. Someone has fallen after being hit by lightning. What severe conditions might you have to treat?

3. You find your neighbour in his garden, unconscious but gripping an electric hedge cutter. Its long cable comes from a first floor window of the house; you cannot get in. Detail your actions.

4. A man carelessly touched a live electric terminal. He says he is pleased that the damage is no more than small dark burn marks on the skin of forefinger and thumb. Why are you less optimistic?

13
Resuscitation

Before you study this chapter please make sure you are familiar with the facts about heart and lungs (pp. 24 and 37).

If suddenly breathing ceases or the heart stops beating (or both) the patient is about to die. After a very few minutes of being deprived of blood flow and of oxygen the brain tissues will die; the nerve control of those functions which keep the body alive will fail.

It can happen in drowning, in choking, in some forms of poisoning and in certain heart attacks. Also electric or lightning shock may sometimes stop the heart. Generally breathing is the first to stop, and failure of the heart beat will follow in a matter of seconds or minutes. The only absolutely reliable signs of the heart's stopping are the patient's sudden loss of consciousness and, at the same time, the fact that an experienced medical person or first aider cannot feel the pulse.

If breathing has stopped you immediately try resuscitation which demands no more than hands and mouth and a little understanding. It has two components:

1. *Artificial Ventilation*—also called Artificial Respiration—and, if necessary:

2. *External Chest Compression*—the name given to pressure on the breastbone to activate the heart pump.

Always begin with Artificial Respiration to fill the lungs with air. Then feel the pulse to check whether the heart is beating and the blood is carrying oxygen from this air through the body and so to the brain. If the pulse is present you know that the patient's heart is working and that his blood is circulating. But you must continue Artificial Ventilation. If the pulse is absent this means that the heart has stopped, and you must add External Chest Compression to the Artificial Ventilation.

These techniques will be described. Learning from the book is certainly possible in the case of Artificial Respiration, but it is far more satisfactory to study and practice in a properly organised first-aid course. As for External Chest Compression this really must be learnt in a course, and you should regard the account given here as a supplement to authorised teaching. In any case *you must never practise on a person, but only on the special manikins provided in the course.*

It is fair to add that the likelihood of having to give resuscitation is not very great. Experts may go for years, or all their lives, without ever meeting the emergency. It is more important to note that, if and when you do meet the emergency, you will have no time for revision and looking-up. You will act without delay and, hopefully, be action perfect because you have learnt meticulously. Then the time you have spent studying could prove its worth by restoring a life.

Has the patient really stopped breathing?

Before beginning any form of artificial ventilation very rapidly make certain that breathing really has stopped. Bend low with your head over the patient's mouth. *Look* sideways for chest movements. *Listen* for air going in and out. Note if you *feel* breaths against your cheek.

Artificial Ventilation

There are three accepted ways of doing this. (1) The *Mouth-to-Mouth method* consists of breathing air from your mouth and lungs into the patient. Undoubtedly it is the most efficient. It is very rare for it to be inoperative and circumstances dictate either (2) the *Holger-Nielsen method* or (3) the *Silvester method*, by which you manipulate the patient's chest so that it alternately contracts and expands, imitating the ordinary breathing movements.

Mouth-to-Mouth

You breathe air from your lungs into that of the patient. Of course your blood will already have absorbed some of the oxygen from that air, but plenty will remain to be of service to the patient. Besides what first passes to the patient as you breathe into him will be air from your mouth and windpipe, air which has not descended into your lungs and therefore has its full oxygen contents. The small amount of carbon dioxide you breathe out of your lungs is too slight to do any harm.

For clarity the steps taken are described in great detail; in fact they can all take place quickly, easily, and smoothly.

1. Rapidly get the patient flat on his back

2. Make sure his throat is not blocked

Give a very, very quick scoop in his mouth with your curved forefinger to clear any possible obstruction— blood, vomit, mud, displaced dentures, etc.

3. Bend his head right back

This makes sure that the tongue is not blocking the airway (p. 49). And you must keep it that way through the whole of resuscitation.

There are several ways of doing this. Lifting the neck by a hand underneath it is not recommended if there is the slightest chance that the patient has hurt the spine in the neck; it could worsen the damage.

The easiest and safest way is to press the head back with the heel of your hand on his forehead with your fingers resting on his nose.

Occasionally these measures are enough; now that his airway is clear the patient begins to breathe spontaneously. If he does not, at once proceed as below.

4. Pinch his nose shut

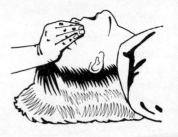

Use the thumb and forefinger of the hand you have on his forehead. This will prevent any air you are about to blow into him from escaping through his nostrils (you will also find that your hold on the nose helps a little to manoeuvre the head back).

Make sure that you pinch the nose correctly by pinching it at its *lower soft part*. Pressing on the upper bony area will not close the nostrils.

5. Make sure his mouth is open

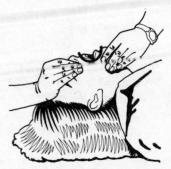

Getting the head back generally makes the mouth fall open. You may have to help it open wider by pulling gently with fingers of your other hand on his chin. Do not let these fingers touch the mouth itself as they would get in the way of your own mouth at the next step.

At the same time you could, if necessary, use your thumb to press the patient's jaw forward. This increases the airway space at the back of the throat in the rare case where bending the head fully back proves insufficient. Be careful that the edge of your hand is not pressing on the front of the patient's neck—a common error.

If you are alone with the patient while you do these important preliminary steps, raise your voice and shout for assistance.

6. Take a deep breath in

7. Seal your mouth round the patient's mouth

Make sure your lips are widely apart, fully covering the opening presented by the patient's mouth.

If the patient has dentures which are in their right position leave them in; they will help to firm his mouth. If the dentures have slipped loose you should quickly remove them.

8. Blow into the patient's mouth

You must not blow harshly for your aim is to fill the lungs as naturally as possible. As you do this, the chest will expand.

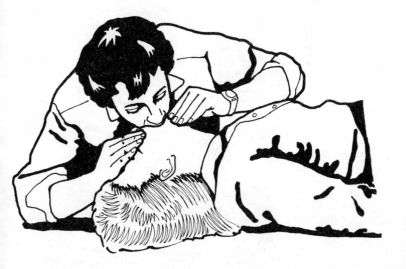

9. *Take your mouth off and let the patient's chest expel air*

It will do this through its natural, elastic recoil. At the same time you take in another breath.

The first four breaths you give very quickly, not waiting for the full flattening of the patient's chest. This puts a high load of oxygen quickly into his lungs.

10. *Try to feel the pulse in the neck*
(p. 25)

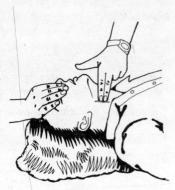

If it is absent you must add External Chest Compression to your endeavours to try to get the circulation going (p. 137).

If it is present then you know that the heart is beating and that blood is carrying the oxygen round the body. You can proceed with step 11.

11. *Maintenance ventilation*

This is the constant repetition of steps 6, 7, 8 and 9. But now your action can be slower.

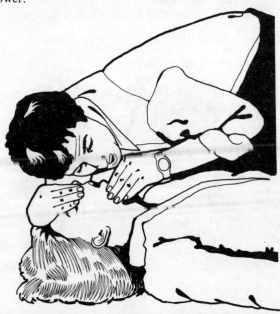

After you have removed your mouth from the patient's face and are taking in another breath keep your head low, looking sideways over the patient's chest. You can verify that it has expanded (i.e. that your blowing had filled the lungs) and that now it is deflating. As soon as the chest has flattened you return to step 7, and so on. This will work out at about 12 to 15 breaths a minute.

Special points about mouth-to-mouth

Emotion

Some people are understandably uneasy about closely mouthing a discovered victim who may be unsavoury. This hesitation has to be overcome. Saving a life is involved.

Unusual positions of the patient

Step 1 tells you to get the patient quickly on his back, but some circumstances may prevent this. It is possible to give mouth-to-mouth to a patient who has to remain in an upright position. It is possible for a strong swimmer rescuing someone in the water to blow into the patient's mouth between strokes. The important thing is to get the first breaths in as soon as possible. On the other hand if someone has been buried under a fall of earth or snow you must get his chest free so that it can expand.

Drowning

In cases of drowning any attempt to tip the patient's head down 'to let water drain out of the lungs' would be a waste of valuable time. Any water which might flow out would be from the windpipe or gullet: its presence there would not interfere with your blown air reaching the lungs.

Interruptions

After any interruption, which may happen, always resume with four quick breaths, to restore a high amount of oxygen.

Vomit

If the patient vomits quickly turn his head to one side and mop out his mouth. Resume ventilation with four quick breaths.

Distended abdomen

The patient's abdomen may become distended because some of the air blown in has bypassed the windpipe and gone down the gullet into the stomach. This is not harmful. But if the distention becomes great it would be a mechanical embarrassment to chest and diaphragm movement. Turn the patient to one side; with one hand gently flatten the upper part of the abdomen to press air up and out; mop away any fluid which comes with it. Then resume Mouth-to-Mouth with four quick breaths.

Problems with chest expansion

If the chest does not expand properly there may still be something wrong with the airway. Check that you are keeping the head back and the nose shut. Make sure your lips are properly placed. If a sense of obstruction remains this could be from choking deep in the airway (see p. 41).

Technique with children

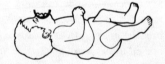

Your lips can seal over both the mouth and the nose of the smaller face. Breathing will be gentler than for an adult—as always just enough to expand the chest. With babies give only little puffs and be careful as you bend the head back; their heads and neck are very pliable and the movement could be overdone.

Your *Maintenance Ventilation* rate will prove a little faster than for the adult: about 20 a minute.

Mouth-to-nose ventilation

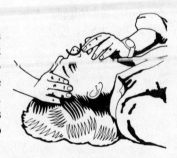

If you cannot use the patient's mouth because it is injured or cannot be kept open, then give Mouth-to-Nose Ventilation. Seal your mouth over the patient's nose, covering both nostrils. Use fingers of one hand to keep his lips well together as you breath into the nose.

The tracheostomy patient

Tracheostomy is an operation which creates a hole in the front of the neck through which the patient breathes. He no longer takes air in through mouth and nose for the hole opens directly into the windpipe. The operation is performed for rare conditions in the upper part of the breathing passage.

Although there are very few people who have had the operation your patient could be one of them. Always give a quick look at the neck as you position him.. If you see the hole (and perhaps a small tube fitted to it) you give Mouth-to-Hole Ventilation instead of Mouth-to-Mouth.

This is straightforward. You do not have to block the nose or do any of the acts to clear mouth and throat. Keep the head straight (but not bent backwards) and seal your mouth around the hole.

External Chest Compression

If the heart is not beating your task is to compress it so that it pumps artificially. An adult's breastbone can be depressed by as much as 5 cm; causing pressure on the heart which lies behind it. This forces out the blood from the heart into the arteries. As soon as the pressure is released the heart fills up again from veins.

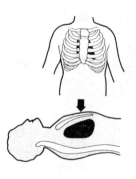

Thus circulation of the blood is artificially created. Of course the action must be repeated rhythmically at the right speed to imitate the heart's natural beat.

1. Get the patient rapidly on to a firm surface

If he is on a soft couch or mattress, pull him carefully to the floor.

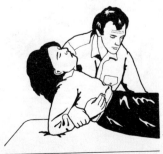

You can help the blood flow to heart and lungs by keeping his legs on the bed or by getting them raised, but do not do this should it delay the next steps.

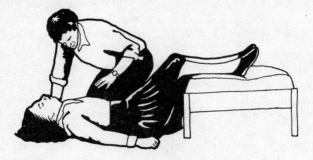

2. Find the point on the breastbone for pressure

The easiest accurate way is to feel the breastbone quickly from top to bottom, to divide its length mentally into thirds and to select the point where the upper two-thirds meet the lower-third.

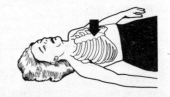

3. Place your hands on the breastbone

Put the heel of one hand on the chosen point and cover it with the heel of the other hand. You must limit your pressure to this point and keep your hands off the rest of the chest.

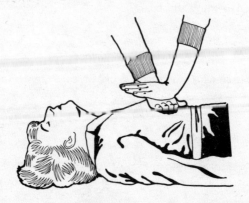

This reduces the risk of damage to ribs or internal organs. Either lock your fingers together or (which is more comfortable) make quite sure that all your fingers are raised off, and remain off, the chest wall.

4. Rock forwards with your arms straight

This is to depress the breastbone 4–5 cm. Do not bend your elbows; do not give a forceful jerk; let the thrust of your body weight do the work.

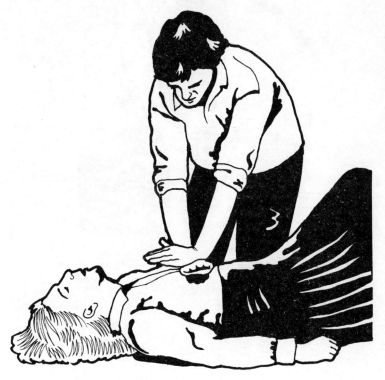

5. Release the compression

Do this as soon as you have made the compression by rocking back. The breastbone will rise again. But do not lift off your hands; the 'heels' of the hands remain in position for the next compression.

6. Repeat steps 4 and 5

These must be repeated rhythmically, to create a blood circulation. But you must also incorporate Artificial Ventilation into your manoeuvres.

When you are working alone

Give 15 Chest Compressions, (at 80 a minute). Then immediately: 2 full Mouth-to-Mouth Ventilations. Then immediately: back to 15 Chest Compressions ... and so on.

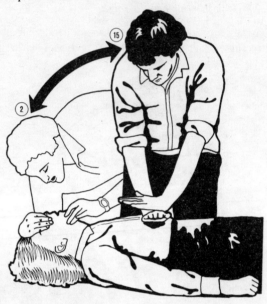

When someone is helping you

If you are the more experienced first aider you will take on the Chest Compressions and, if necessary, instruct your helper to do the

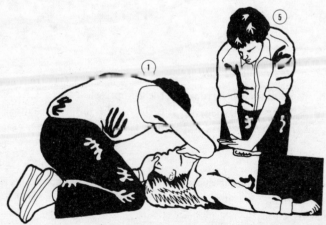

ventilations. If possible, you and your helper will be on opposite sides of the patient so as not to get in each other's way.

Give Chest Compressions at the rate of 60 a minute (1 a second).

At the upstroke of every fifth compression your helper (who has been carefully watching and counting) gives one full Mouth-to-Mouth Ventilation. (You do not interrupt your Chest Compressions while he ventilates; carry on without pause.)

Technique with children

Use much less force and slightly greater speed for Chest Compression of children.

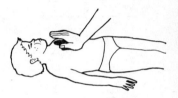

The heel of one hand on the breastbone is enough for the average child.

For a small baby press lightly with only a couple of fingers on the *centre* of the breastbone. This is a relatively higher position than in the adult because the baby's large liver takes up so much space in the lower part of the chest.

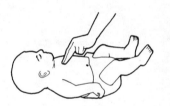

Increase the speed to 100 a minute to fit in with the normally faster heart beat of children. But the proportion of Chest Compressions to ventilations remains the same as for the adult: 15 to 2 (one first aider) or 5 to 1 (two first aiders).

Check as you Go

Combined Chest Compression and Artificial Ventilation aim to get the heart beating and the chest breathing spontaneously again. Unless you test you will not know how successful your resuscitating is. Furthermore it is harmful to give Chest Compression when the heart is already beating at its own rhythm.

Therefore you should make regular checks. As already described you feel for the neck pulse after the first four quick ventilations. If they are absent, you add Chest Compression to your efforts. One minute later feel again for the spontaneous pulse. Thereafter, if necessary, you check every three minutes for its return.

The Patient is not breathing

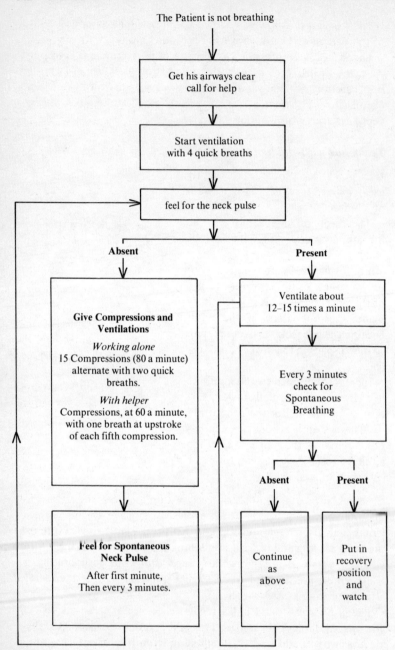

Get his airways clear
call for help

Start ventilation
with 4 quick breaths

feel for the neck pulse

Absent   **Present**

**Give Compressions and
Ventilations**

Working alone
15 Compressions (80 a minute)
alternate with two quick
breaths.

With helper
Compressions, at 60 a minute,
with one breath at upstroke
of each fifth compression.

Ventilate about
12–15 times a minute

Every 3 minutes
check for
Spontaneous
Breathing

Absent   **Present**

**Feel for Spontaneous
Neck Pulse**

After first minute,
Then every 3 minutes.

Continue
as
above

Put in
recovery
position
and
watch

SEND TO HOSPITAL BY
AMBULANCE AS SOON
AS POSSIBLE.

If you find that there is pulsation in the neck artery, then the heart is beating and you should not begin or pursue further the Chest Compression. Continue Artificial Ventilation as long as there is no spontaneous breathing. Also make a quick check of the pulse every three minutes to reassure yourself the heart is still beating.

With success the patient's own spontaneous breathing will also return. This too you should look for every three minutes. As they begin again the chest movements may be slight and uneven and you will have to help them, adapting your Mouth-to-Mouth Ventilation to keep in time with them.

When spontaneous breathing is stronger and regular you can stop the Mouth-to-Mouth Ventilation.

Now put the patient in the Recovery Position (p. 112) and keep on checking his pulse and breathing in case they fail again.

How Long Should Attempts Continue?

In theory you continue until the patient recovers. This has been known to happen after several hours of resuscitation attempts. Carry on without interruption and use bystanders to help by sending urgent messages for aid and ambulance, by loosening tight clothes and by covering the patient lightly with blankets. (But do not have the chest obscured.)

If there is no apparent recovery, continue until someone experienced and of authority (essentially a doctor) advises you to desist.

A first aider who has correctly tried resuscitation but has not succeeded will feel very disappointed. But he should not be discouraged. Many patients whose heart beat and respiration stop can never recover. This cannot be foretold at the onset of the incident. First aiders must try resuscitation at once, well aware that, in only a proportion of cases, can they achieve the privilege of saving a life. When it does happen the event is marvellously memorable.

Risks of Resuscitation

Blowing too hard

This could damage the patient's lungs. This is particularly true when dealing with babies and small children. Mouth-to-Mouth breathing should be enough to expand and raise the patient's chest, but no harder.

Pressing too hard on the chest

This may injure bones or the organs underlying them, especially in the elderly whose chest walls have relatively poor resilience, and in babies who need very little pressure.

Avoid injury by not bending your elbows and by not lunging.

Pressing too widely on the chest

Pressing should be restricted to one point on the breastbone. By extending beyond this it could crack ribs or damage organs like liver, lungs or even heart. Keep your fingers locked together or off the chest wall.

'Resuscitating' unnecessarily

Many ill-informed people rush to 'resuscitate' anyone who collapses and falls, without making sure that respiration, and perhaps heart beat, have ceased.

Never try artificial ventilation or chest compression when heart and lungs are still functioning of their own accord. You could do great harm.

Medical attention is always needed

If you have resuscitated successfully do not merely rejoice and leave it at that. Your patient should be checked by a doctor, preferably after ambulance transport to hospital.

Mouth-to-mouth artificial ventilation and infection

When practising on a model

Cleaning the contact area with any efficient antiseptic between individual use is perfectly adequate to prevent infection.

When resuscitating someone

There is no valid evidence that the virus of a severe infection (e.g. AIDS) can be transmitted to the rescuer. The risk is considered to be so extremely remote that first aiders should proceed without hesitation.

Other Methods of Artificial Ventilation

The Mouth-to-Mouth method is the best. It is rare not to be able to use it. A patient may have serious facial injuries. He may be repeatedly vomiting; this could cause him to choke were he to be kept on his back. He might be pinned down, face downwards or have injuries which preclude turning him on his back. He might have taken a strong poison whose traces, about his mouth, could endanger the first aider.

Two alternative techniques use the principle of manipulating the patient's chest to narrow and then widen it, so that air is expelled from and drawn into the lungs. Both methods include pressure by the first aider: *this pressure is quite different from that used for acting on the heart.*

Holger-Nielsen Method

It is named after the Danish army medical officer who described it in 1932.

1. Quickly clear the mouth of any obstruction

This is as described for the Mouth-to-Mouth method.

2. Position the patient rapidly

The position is on the ground, face downwards. Turn his head sideways and bent back. Tuck his two hands, one above the other, under his head so that his cheek rests on them.

3. Quickly position your hands

Kneel on one knee close to and in front of the patient. Place your hands over his upper back so that your wrists lie level with an imaginary line between the top of his armpits, and your thumbs on either side of the backbone. Spread your palms and fingers over the shoulder blades.

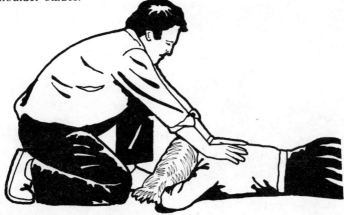

4. Keeping your arms straight, rock forwards steadily

Do this until your arms are about vertical. The weight of your body presses through your arms on the patient's upper back. You do not push with your arms. This step takes two seconds. By compressing the chest, it expels air from the lungs.

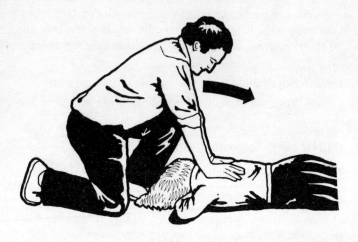

5. Rock backwards and release the pressure

As you do so slide your hands off the patient's back and along the outer side of his arms to grasp them just above the elbows. Let this point be reached well before you complete rocking back. Now as you rock back further your straight arms will lift the patient's elbows.

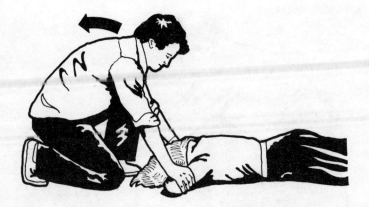

This step widens the patient's chest and draws air into his lungs: it takes three seconds.

A common mistake is getting the hands to their positions near the patient's elbows before completing the rocking back. This would mean that the first aider now has to pull with his shoulder muscles instead of just letting the swing of his arms do the work. It is less efficient, and quite tiring.

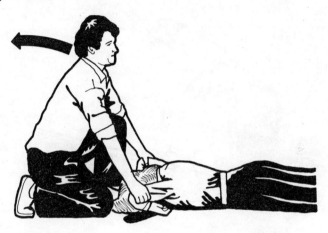

6. *Return to your first position*

Quickly lower the patient's elbows and slide your hands back over the shoulder blades as you bend forward again.

Now repeat steps 4, 5, and 6. Together they should take about 5 seconds.

Do 4 such cycles and then feel for the patient's neck pulse. If it is present, carry on with this method.

If it is absent you must try to get the heart beating by External Chest Compression on the breast bone as already described (p. 137). This means having to turn the patient on his back. And that will mean having now to use the Silvester Method for Artificial Ventilation. Why then does one not use the Silvester Method at the onset? The reason is that tests have shown how, when the patient's heart is beating, the Holger-Nielsen gives better artificial ventilation than the Silvester.

Silvester Method

This is named after an English doctor who described it in 1861.

1. Quickly clear the mouth of any obstruction

This is as described for the Mouth-to-Mouth method.

2. Position the patient rapidly

Get him on his back. Push a firm thick pad (cushion, folded coat or blanket) well under his shoulders so that you can bend the head back-

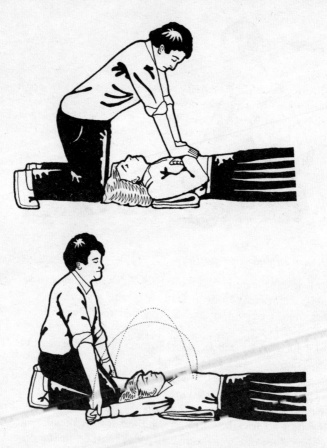

wards to ensure that the tongue is not blocking the throat. A common error is to put the pad too high under the neck instead of the shoulders.

3. Position yourself rapidly

Kneel at the patient's head. With each hand grasp one of the patient's wrists and cross them over the lower part of his chest.

4. Keeping your arms straight, rock forwards steadily

Do this until your arms are about vertical. The weight of your body presses through your arms on the patient's chest. You do not push with your arms.

This step takes two seconds. By compressing the chest, it expels air from the lungs.

5. Rock backwards and release the pressure

Still holding the patient's wrists, you sweep his arms in a wide arc up and outwards and then downwards until they are nearly on the ground.

This step takes three seconds. It widens the patient's chest and draws air into his lungs. The movement you give to the patient is comparable to the action of someone who, on getting up, stretches his arm up and outwards with a deep breath to invigorate himself.

6. Return to your first position

Now repeat steps 4, 5, and 6. Together they should take about 5 seconds. Do 4 such cycles and then feel for the patient's neck pulse. If it is present, carry on with this method. If it is absent, you must try to get the heart beating by External Chest Compression on the breastbone as already described (p. 00). Alternate 15 breastbone pressure with 2 cycles of Artificial Ventilation.

Questions

1. Before giving Mouth-to-Mouth Ventilation how do you ensure that the air blown into the patient's mouth will reach his lungs? And after blowing how do you confirm that this has happened?

2. A middle-aged woman, in front of you in a supermarket, suddenly falls to the ground and lies motionless. From the other end of the store the manager calls for someone to resuscitate her. What do you do?

3. Of the three methods of Artificial Ventilation described in this chapter the Silvester is considered the least effective. When and why should one use it?

4. Both Mouth-to-Mouth Ventilation and the Holger-Nielsen method aim to get air into the patient's lungs. Describe how each achieves this in a different way.

5. A dumper truck tips a large load of sand accidentally knocking down and fully covering a man. His mate has quickly cleared his face. What do you do now?

6. You are called to the bedside of a man who, quite suddenly, has stopped breathing. After beginning Artificial Ventilation you find there is no pulse in the neck. Detail your next actions.

14
Foreign Bodies

Objects in the Wrong Place

'Foreign body' is a doctor's term for an object which has become lodged in an abnormal place of the body. The wound with an object embedded in it is dealt with on p. 4.

Splinters

Clean the area around the splinter with soap and water before you examine it.

If part of the splinter is projecting you may try to use fine tweezers. Sterilise them first by boiling in water for ten minutes. (Do not hold the tips in a match flame for this is likely to coat them with a sooty deposit.) Rest the part of the body with the splinter on a firm surface in a good light. Clean the skin area with swab and water or an accurately diluted antiseptic. Once the forceps have been sterilised do not let their tips touch anything but the skin area concerned. Grasp the splinter as near the skin as possible and pull it out gently.

Wooden splinters often break, leaving a segment under the skin. If this happens, or if the splinter is totally embedded, you proceed no further and let a doctor or nurse deal with it. In any case medical advice is needed to cover the risk of infection (including tetanus).

Fish Hooks

When only the point has entered the skin the hook can be pulled out. If it has moved deeper, so that the barb has penetrated, pulling on it would cause pain and laceration. The problem should be brought to a doctor as soon as possible. Meantime put padding around the hook so that it will

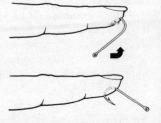

not move and bandage carefully over
this.

It may happen that, because medical help will not be available, you
have to get the hook out yourself.
Begin by washing the hook and skin
area very gently. Push the hook in
further, turning its shaft so that the
barb now comes out through a
separate hole. Steadying the hook,
cut off the barb. Now pull out the
remainder of the hook, reversing the
path used when you pushed it in.
Clean the skin and dress the wound.
You must refer the patient to a doctor
for the risk of infection (including
tetanus) is high.

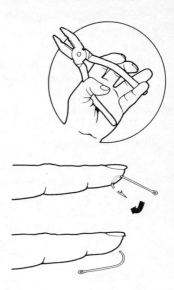

In the Nose

Children, with their experimental curiosity, are the likely patients,
having pushed something like a pebble or a bean up one nostril. Beans
absorb moisture, swell and become very difficult to displace.

Do not try to probe the object out yourself. You may push it in
further and also hurt the inside of the nose. The doctor or the nurse has
the right apparatus for visualising and extracting the object.

The most that could be done by the patient is one, very gentle, nose
blowing. If (as is likely) this does not succeed he should persist no
further.

In the Ear

As with an object in the nose, you
should not try to probe it out; this
would risk damaging the ear drum.
Let the patient consult a doctor or a
nurse.

An insect in the ear however you
may deal with, especially as its lively
movements can be intensely unpleasant to the patient. Let him lie or
bend his head with the ear uppermost.
With one hand hold the top of the

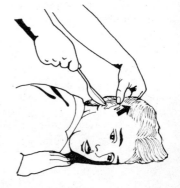

outer ear pulling it upwards and backwards; this straightens the ear canal, which normally is slightly kinked. With the other hand pour in a little water (preferably tepid, but not hot) into the canal. The insect will float to the top and can be wiped away.

But you must not try this if the patient is known or suspected to have a damaged ear drum. Water might pass beyond it and harm the deeper parts of the ear.

Swallowed Objects

From marbles to safety pins—all sorts of objects may be swallowed by mistake. This is a matter mainly for reassurance, and not for first aid. Most of them, even the sharp ones, will give little or no trouble. They will move along the bowel to be passed out in due course. A doctor should be consulted if there is any doubt. Certainly you should not give purgatives or think of trying to make the patient vomit.

The same may be said about fish bones stuck at the back of the throat. Painful as they may be, they are best left for medical help. Many will come out of their own accord.

In the Eye

(Wounds of the eye: p. 5. Chemicals in the eye: p. 98.)

A piece of grit or small particle, which gets on the eyeball, generally sets the patient blinking and rubbing, which makes it move to lie under one or other lid. The first thing to do is to advise the patient to stop rubbing. Then try, in turn, the following steps.

1. Let the patient blink in a basin of clean water. This is worth trying for its simplicity, but it does not often succeed in getting the object out.

2. Wash your hands. Sit the patient down in a good light and stand behind him. Let him bend his head back as you look down. Ask him to relax for probably he is keeping the eye firmly shut. Gently separate the lids and survey the eye all over while he moves it slowly in all directions.

3. If you see the object on the white of the eye try to pick it off with a moistened twisted tip of a clean handkerchief. Do not try more than twice If it does not come away it is likely to be not just lying on but firmly embedded in the surface of the eye. Then you must put a soft pad over the eye and send the patient to a doctor or to hospital.

4. *If the object is anywhere within the coloured circle of the eye leave it alone.* It is on the area through which light enters and must be

dealt with by a doctor, since first-aid handling could leave a scar. Limit yourself to covering the eye with a soft pad.

5. If the object is not visible on the front of the eye now look under the lower lid, pulling it gently and fully down while the patient *looks upward*. Use the moist handkerchief tip to lift away the object.

6. However, usually the object lies beneath the upper lid. If the previous step has not shown it, you must finally look for it there. Hold

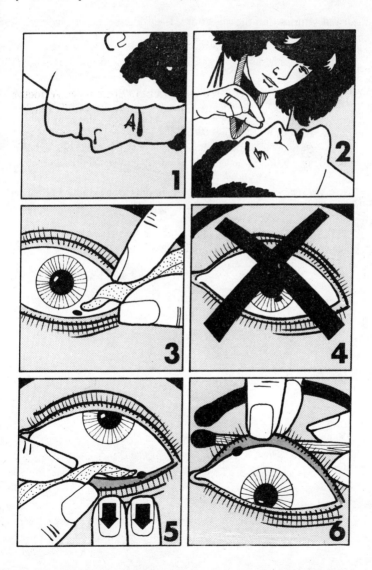

a matchstick along the 'hinge' of the lid, with its rounded end against the nose. Ask the patient to *look down*. Take the edge of the lid between finger and thumb and evert it over the matchstick. A firm grasp by you feels easier to the patient and is more likely to succeed than a light one. Use the moist handkerchief tip to lift away the object.

The manoeuvre may seem awkward for the first aider and uncomfortable for the patient, but those who have experienced it find it very acceptable.

7. If you cannot find the object or if the eye appears very red, apply a soft pad and send the patient to a doctor.

Questions

1. Billy, aged five, has, by mistake, swallowed a small toy brick, which he had been sucking. He is tearful and so is his mother. What help can you give?

2. Someone on the river bank has managed to extract a fish hook from an angler's ear. There is no bleeding. What advice do you give?

3. Describe what you would do about a small piece of grit in someone's eye: (a) below the upper lid; (b) on the white area; (c) on the coloured ring of the iris.

4. Near the tent where you are camping on the moors, you find an angler with a fish hook deeply embedded in the thumb. (He is fifty miles from home, having come by car.) What do you do?

5. A friend asks for help for her boy, aged 14. His ear is recovering from a deep infection (with temporary deafness and discharge) but now is bothered by an insect inside it. How do you act?

15
The Poisoned Patient

In the past, first-aid treatment for poisoning laid stress on making the patient vomit and on giving 'antidotes'. Today these measures have been largely discarded outside hospitals. In any case there are very few real antidotes, that is drugs which will specifically counter a poison.

Today first aid aims to safeguard the patient's breathing and to get him as rapidly as possible to hospital for specialised care.

The Path of the Poison

The word 'poison' suggests a toxic substance *swallowed* by accident or, in suicide or criminal cases, by design. But many medicines and chemicals, harmless or useful in ordinary doses, become poisonous in abnormally large amounts.

Also there are several ways in which the poison can enter and harm the body. Some swallowed substances will do local damage to lips, mouth, throat, gullet, and stomach. They then will be absorbed into the blood stream which carries them to act nefariously on special organs like brain, nerves, heart, kidneys or liver. A few will interfere with the life-protecting powers of the blood cells.

A poison can enter direct into the lungs as a gas, as particles in fumes or as fine droplets *in the air breathed in*. There are also substances, like sprays of certain horticulturally-used chemicals, which can be *absorbed through the skin* into the body. And finally some poisons can be *injected* directly into the body; these include the venom of snakes (p. 165) and the dangerous preparations self-administered by drug addicts.

First-Aid Measures

If you are called to a case of poisoning, this is your routine.

1. Check whether the patient is conscious or unconscious

Touch him and talk to him.

2. *If he is unconscious check whether he is breathing*

Look for chest movements; with your head near his mouth listen and feel for air moving in and out.

If there appear to be breathing difficulties his airway may be blocked; act as described on p. 46 to clear the airway.

If he is breathing properly (and has no injury which precludes your moving him) put him in the Recovery Position (p. 112).

If he is not breathing begin Resuscitation at once (p. 130). Some drugs like morphia can, in abnormally large doses, interfere with the brain's ability to maintain respiration.

For another reason you should also rapidly find out what the patient took. Look at any poison container by him or ask bystanders. In some rare cases of poisons like cyanide (Prussic Acid) you must avoid contaminating yourself; do not use the Mouth-to-Mouth method of artificial respiration but turn to the Holger-Nielsen method.

3. *If he is conscious ask the patient what he took*

Get a story from him at once lest later he becomes unconscious.

4. *Send immediately for an ambulance*

It is generally better to do this than to call a doctor since he may not be immediately reachable. And at this stage the doctor himself could do little more than could the good first aider and the ambulance staff.

5. *Give the conscious patient bland drinks*

Most poisons inflame the lining of the stomach; diluting them reduces this effect. Giving much fluid could encourage the breaking-up of capsules or tablets, which had been swallowed whole, and thereby hasten their absorption into the patient's system. On the other hand a high concentration of poison against the stomach lining can be extremely damaging and can itself hasten absorption. On balance diluting the poison is necessary.

You may give water or barley water but the best drink would be milk whose physical properties can 'bind' the poison to it and so delay absorption.

The amount you give is about two tumblerfuls, to be taken slowly. If possible, and easy, give it tepid (not hot) but not if this means wasting time heating it.

You will never try to give anything to drink to someone who is unconscious or too drowsy to swallow. The fluid would enter his windpipe and choke him.

6. *Put the patient in the Recovery Position (p. 112)*

Afterwards cover him loosely and await the ambulance.

(There is an old and quite false idea that someone who has taken an overdose of sedative or sleeping tablets should be forced to walk about. This would only fail and could prove harmful. The patient must be at rest.)

7. *Observation*

While waiting always watch the patient closely. At any point a conscious patient may become unconscious or a breathing patient may cease breathing and need Resuscitation.

Someone who has made a suicide attempt must remain under careful observation. He may seek to make another attempt by some desperate action like jumping out of a high window.

Another thing to do while waiting is to collect any evidence of the poison taken by the patient: containers, medicine bottles or pill boxes. Hand these to the ambulance attendants to take to hospital; even if they are empty their labels may give valuable information. If the patient has vomited spontaneously send a sample of the vomit in a clean container; label this and add your estimate of the total amount the patient did bring up.

If there is time you should send a telephone message to the emergency department of the hospital to announce the imminent arrival of the patient and to tell what you believe the poison to be.

Should One try to Make the Patient Vomit?

Almost always the answer to this is a clear '**NO**'. First-aid attempts to make the patient vomit have sometimes led to unfortunate complications. You should instead concentrate on protecting the patient's airway and getting him to hospital quickly.

In a few, very unusual, circumstances a case could be made for inducing vomiting. If the patient is really far from medical help it would be reasonable to try to get the poison out of his stomach.

But you should not try to induce vomiting unless **all** (not just some) of the following conditions apply:

(a) It will take more than a couple of hours to get the patient to hospital.

(b) The attempt will in no way delay the call for an ambulance.

(c) The patient is fully conscious.

(d) He is fully co-operative, and can sit up and bend over a basin.

(e) He has been given the bland drinks described above.

(f) The poison taken is **not** petrol, gasoline, kerosene paraffin, turpentine or a similar product. When they are being swallowed these volatile substances produce vapours which move down the windpipe. They will cause severe damage to the lungs. Were the patient to vomit then vapours would again have access to the windpipe and the harm would increase.

(g) The poison taken is **not** a corrosive, e.g. acid, caustic soda, ammonia or bleach. They severely burn the areas between lips and stomach through which they pass. If vomited they would burn them further. Also the corroded stomach or gullet walls could perforate during the strong contractile actions of vomiting. Then the poison would pass out of the stomach to enter and to burn the general space of the abdomen or chest and the other organs within it.

(h) You do not induce vomiting by giving any substance like salt (which has proved to be, not only inefficient but also potentially dangerous). The only method you should use is that of touching the back of the patient's throat, while he is ready to bend forward and vomit. This can be done with one or two fingers or with the blunt handle of a spoon around which you have wrapped a cloth.

The teaching is repeated: do **not** try to make the patient vomit except in the rare circumstance when **all** the conditions above co-exist.

Corrosive Poisons

Acids, strong alkalis, liquids like caustic soda, ammonia and bleach will burn the mouth and lips very painfully and are likely to stain around the mouth. Let the patient have plenty of fluid (water or milk) to rinse out these parts. Clean any splashes away from the skin and check that none has entered the eyes (see p. 98).

Garden and Agricultural Poisons

Some of the chemicals used as pesticides and as weedkillers can be extremely harmful to man. Their use is governed by strict advice and safety regulations. If these are disregarded the user can become poisoned.

Fine sprays, wind-borne, may be breathed in. Or they may settle on clothes and skin, from which they pass into the body. The effect of strong concentrations will be rapid. But the effect of sustained weaker

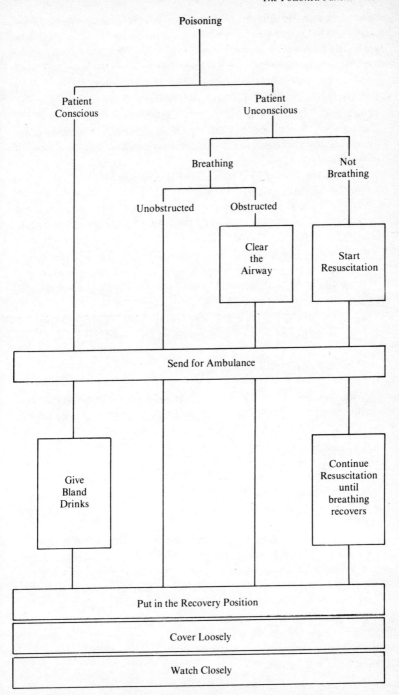

exposures may be delayed and cumulative. The poison can build up relatively slowly in a patient who would, over hours, or even days, only gradually develop symptoms.

Initially the symptoms may be slight. Certain pesticides will produce the following: headache, abnormal sweating, thirst, feeling hot with general aching. The appetite is poor and the patient may feel, or be, sick. Then he experiences muscle weakness, and action of the chest muscles is reduced, so that breathing is difficult. Vision becomes dim. This could progress to coma and to convulsing, and to failure of respiration.

With anyone using such chemicals suspect poisoning as soon as he begins to feel 'out-of-sorts'.

1. Get him away from the area of work and put him at complete rest.
2. Remove any contaminated clothes. If possible put them in a plastic bag, taking care not to contaminate yourself; wear gloves.
3. Wash his skin thoroughly and include washing out the eyes (p. 98).
4. If his skin is very hot and dry sponge him with cold water.
5. Give drinks of milk or water, with added sugar and a small pinch of salt.
6. Send for an ambulance.

Some containers of these chemicals have labels or accompanying leaflets with useful specific advice on action if poisoning is suspected.

Poisoning by Plants

The principal victims are small children who like to try eating attractive berries or leaves. Remember that they may experiment this way and keep the fact secret from adults even when they begin to feel the ill-effects.

Mushrooms are always a risk for those who are not absolute experts on which are edible. Some mushrooms are always poisonous; some only at certain phases of their development; some only if eaten raw. None of the myths about testing the mushroom by its darkening effect on silver or by the ease of peeling it are any use as a guide to safety.

Symptoms (vomiting, diarrhoea, collapse and sometimes convulsions) may appear in a few minutes with certain mushrooms, but with the majority they are delayed from two to twenty-four hours after they have been eaten.

Food Poisoning

See p. 199.

Alcohol

In large amounts alcohol is a potent poison and has been the cause of many deaths. If you find someone unconscious or nearing unconsciousness do not let an odour of alcohol about him reassure you that he is 'only drunk'. Take all the necessary measures for unconsciousness (p. 110) including safeguarding the airway, seeing to the Recovery Position (p. 112), and keep a careful watch.

Alcohol in conjunction with sedatives or sleeping tablets is particularly dangerous. Each increases the effect of the other. Large, but still safe, doses of either can be lethal when taken in combination.

Carbon Monoxide

In Britain, North Sea gas, which is non-toxic, has superseded coal gas which is poisonous because of the carbon monoxide it contains.

Do not confuse the harmful carbon *mon*oxide with the non-poisonous carbon *dio*xide, which is formed by the body tissues as they use oxygen in their life processes (p. 37) and is also a product of anything that burns. If carbon monoxide is breathed into the lungs it passes to the blood, and there it links on to the chemicals of the red blood cells. In doing this it blocks the red cells' power to take in oxygen. The circulating blood can no longer transport oxygen effectively round the body, and the patient may die from oxygen lack.

Carbon monoxide may be formed by the engine of a motor car running with the throttle fully open. If this happens in a closed garage the motorist may be poisoned. Another source of this gas could be any fire in a room with little or no ventilation. At first the fire turns oxygen present into carbon dioxide in the ordinary and harmless way. As oxygen is used up and not replaced by incoming fresh air, the burning produces carbon monoxide instead. Accidents of this sort can happen where flues are inadequate or where someone has tried to keep out the cold by blocking door and windows against draughts and using some form of fire to warm himself.

A high concentration of carbon monoxide can be rapidly fatal. But most cases of the poisoning happen through a gradual increase of the gas in the atmosphere. Then symptoms develop insidiously: headache, noises in the ears, dizziness and nausea. Muscle weakness follows to an extent that by the time the victim realises something is amiss he is unable to move or call out. The complexion of the poisoned man may be abnormally red, but more often is grey and blue-tinged.

Rescue from a room full of dangerous gas fumes is described on p. 92. Where carbon monoxide (which is colourless and odourless) is suspected, the rescuer should wear an oxygen mask unless he can move very rapidly in, and out, while holding his breath.

If Preventable, Why not Prevented?

Almost all of this chapter relates to disasters that need never happen. And yet hospitals daily receive poisoning cases caused mainly by lack of care. It is well worth listing some of the simple home precautions, which could, and should, be taken. Many of them are based on the fact that most poisoning happens to unguarded small children who cannot distinguish pills from sweets and whose palates are ready to try anything.

Home Medicine Cabinet

This should be of difficult access to children and of the safety type needing two hands to open it. Keep medicines to be used externally (e.g. liniments) apart from those to be swallowed. However familiar the container appears, always read the label before taking the dose. Discard left-over medication down the lavatory.

Bedroom

Do not keep pills or medicines by the bedside. Put cosmetics, nail varnish and perfume out of children's reach.

Kitchen

Have high shelves and cupboards to hold things like polishes, detergents, turpentine, disinfectants, bleaches, fabric conditioners, and oven cleaners.

Pantry

This should hold only food.

Garden

Keep all horticultural chemicals on high shelves in a locked shed. Teach children to leave plants alone and that what can be eaten by birds and animals is not necessarily safe for them.

Garage

Place antifreeze, cleaners and other chemicals on a high shelf. Make petrol cans inaccessible. Do not keep the car running in the garage.

In general

No handbag should hold more than the day's dose of any medication. Make sure all bottles are accurately labelled. Never pour a liquid usually kept in a characteristically-shaped bottle (e.g. disinfectant) into another whose shape suggests a drinkable liquid (e.g. wine).

The Drug Addict

The causes of and the general state of addiction are matters not for first aid but for long and painstaking medical and social help. However, an addict may go into acute crises with which you have to deal immediately.

Sudden collapse, convulsions or unconsciousness

You deal with this according to the general first-aid help to poisoning and to epilepsy (pp. 155, 193).

Deep depression

This can motivate a suicidal act. Remain with the patient to protect him. Discuss sympathetically and constructively any matters he will talk about.

Overactivity and excitement

Deal with him as if he were drunk. Talk with him all the time in a friendly way and aim to remain on good terms. Stay with him until he calms down or you can get help.

Hallucinations

These may be the most difficult to manage. The patient can have extraordinary ideas of power, like being able to leap from a dangerous height. Or he may be in a panic, convinced that he will be attacked and must retaliate. Reassure him as best you can; try to appear calm and settled in contrast to his behaviour; try to redirect his interest; speak comfortingly. Constantly watch for your own safety; use force only as needed to safeguard yourself and him. Seek help rapidly. In severe cases ambulance transport to hospital is necessary.

In none of your actions should you censure the patient or show him signs of despair. He must get a chance to feel that you wish him well and can help.

Questions

1. During the second day of busily spraying his orchard near your home, an acquaintance comes to request aspirin and a drink of water. He feels thirsty, tired and aching and thinks he may be starting influenza. Describe how best you can help him.

2. On a warm summer's day you find a tramp, breathing noisily and unrousable, on the flowerbed of a local park. Two empty bottles of 'British Vodka' lie near him. Should you interfere and, if so, how? Should you notify anyone—and, if so, whom?

3. A two-year old runs in with a bottle she found in the room next door and cries cheerfully: 'All gone, Mummy!'. The bottle, now empty, held camphorated oil. What should her mother do?

4. A small group in a foreign mountain trek is one day distant from the nearest native village. An hour after eating unknown berries one man goes pale and sweating with severe stomach pains. He wants to carry on, and the group leader decides ... what?

5. Do you agree that the illustration below is a good tribute to the parental care in the home? Explain your answer in detail.

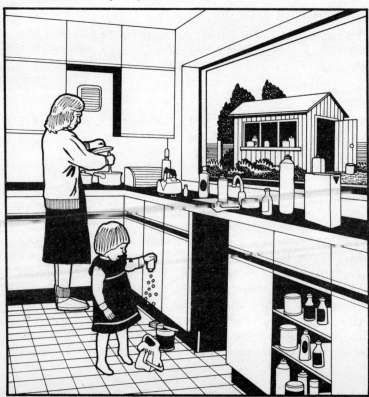

16
Animals and Plants

Animal Bites

Treat them as you would any wound (p. 1). Remember that these carry a high risk of infection and, in particular, that of tetanus. Always tell the patient to consult his doctor for advice after such injuries.

Rabies is a very unlikely risk in Britain, a country protected by the sea and by strict regulations which govern the way animals can be imported. But the danger does exist in many other countries, and it is not restricted to 'mad dogs'. The virus can live in any warm-blooded animal and be transmitted through its saliva. Dogs, cats, foxes and bats can be victims and can spread the disease. The animal may appear normal at the time or may suggestively behave in an enraged manner, attacking man without provocation.

If there is any suspicion that the patient has been bitten by a rabid animal:

1. Wash the wound immediately and thoroughly with soap and water, not hesitating to use a scrubbing brush.
2. Send the patient to a doctor.
3. If possible get the attacking animal isolated and seen by a veterinary surgeon.
4. Notify the police.

Snakebite

In Britain the only poisonous snake is the adder. Fortunately it is relatively harmless. Although its bite can cause intense pain and, in serious cases, collapse it is very rare for it to be fatal—except to the very young or elderly and to those with severe heart trouble.

The adder, about 60 cm (24 in.) long is a tough-looking snake. Colour varies from yellow to orange-brown, and the dark markings are striking. A wide zigzag runs along the back and the sides bear

rough blotches; there is also a prominent X mark at the top of the head.
This head is characteristically club-
shaped, broadening from the body.

In contrast Britain's other two
common snakes are quite harmless.
They have a slighter and streamlined
shape with finer markings. The
Smooth Snake is of the same length
as the adder but slimmer. Its colour is
grey or brown and its markings
restricted to a paired series of small
spots on the back. The *Grass Snake* is
a metre (40 in.) or more in length and
its colour is like the adder's. It too has
small, paired spots on the back, with
as well, some vertical bars on the side.

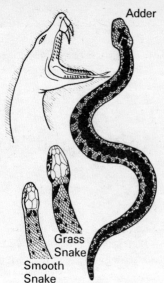

Adder

Grass
Snake

Smooth
Snake

Adders are feared more than they merit. They reserve offensive
attacks for food, like voles or mice. Attacks on men are defensive, i.e.
when they are disturbed and frightened. The victim may have walked
on or near an adder in long grass, or have brushed a hedge, or moved a
pile of stones or logs, which hid it.

The adder can strike from a distance of 30 cm (1 ft). As it opens its
mouth it will swing out and expose two hollow fangs, which pierce the
victim's skin; the poison is injected as from syringe needles. Then the
snake is likely to slither away, out of sight, with speed. Such events are
more likely in the warm weather of summer.

Two puncture marks, 1 cm apart, show in the skin. Sometimes only
one fang penetrates leaving a single mark. Pain, swelling and redness
are likely to develop quickly. More general effects may develop within
two hours: sweating, nausea, vomiting, dizziness and a feeling of
collapse. (Sometimes however such symptoms arise emotionally from
the patient's anxiety.) Breathing may become weak and (rarely) even
fail. The later effects of the poison could include weakening of the
heart beat. Interference with blood clotting may show as bruise spots.

In the majority of cases symptoms are much less severe, especially if
the adder has not been able to empty a full dose of poison through its
fangs.

Treatment of Adder Bites

1. Reassurance

This is fully justified and often necessary. The bitten patient is likely to be extremely frightened. Tell him firmly that he will survive, even if he does feel bad pain and distress.

2. Wipe or wash away

Use soap and water to remove any drops of poison lying on the skin.

3. Remove any possibly constricting object

This includes objects like a ring from the bitten area before swelling develops.

4. Immobilise the bitten part

Restricting its movement decreases the blood circulation within it and therefore reduces dissemination of the poison from it. Your aim is to slow the spread of the poison into the rest of the body as much as possible.

Put the patient at rest, lying down and treat the bitten part as if it were fractured. Keep it as low as possible. Take general anti-shock measures (p. 105).

5. Cover the bite area with a clean dressing

Let the dressing include a thick pad and wide bandage—which you may have to improvise (p. 12). Firmness (not tightness) of the bandage over the pad, by compressing the skin and its blood vessels, contributes to decreasing the circulation in that area. Please note that this is **not** a tourniquet—a thing you should **not** use.

6. Give pain relief tablets with water

If you have them and if the patient is conscious and can swallow. Let him take them before the pain builds up fully. In this case paracetamol tablets are better than aspirin since the latter could possibly aggravate the blood-damaging effect of the poison. Also encourage the patient to drink water or a non-alcoholic liquid like tea copiously but frequently in small amounts (for this reduces the likelihood of vomiting).

This is one of the rare occasions when it is correct to break the general first-aid rule, i.e. not giving the patient anything by mouth.

Anyone who is alone when bitten should make for a place where he can get help, walking slowly and taking frequent rests.

7. *Transport the patient to hospital*

Do this as rapidly as possible. Try to keep him in the Recovery Position with the bitten limb hanging down. Watch him in case he vomits or in case he stops breathing and needs Resuscitation.

If (which is unlikely) you have managed to kill the snake take the body with you to hospital for identification. But you must be careful since even after death the head may bite reflexly when touched. Handle it only with a long stick.

Warning

Do not use a tourniquet (tight band round a limb). Do not apply potassium permanganate crystals. Do not apply ice. Do not suck the wound. Do not cut the wound. All these measures have been advocated in the past, but are inappropriate and possibly dangerous in adder bites.

Other Venomous Snakes

Some people keep pet snakes from overseas which are said to be 'harmless' until one day they strike and poison. Venomous snakes are found in zoos. All over the world, snakes abound, notably in Africa, India, Arabia, and the United States. When they strike, first aid follows the same lines as described above for the adder in Britain. Speed of transport to medical care is very important.

In some of these cases local experts advise suction to the bite or lightly constrictive bands on a limb just above the wound or firm bandaging (as for a sprain) to the limb, or small superficial incisions to the wound. Conditions of poisoning vary so greatly in different places and with different snakes that you should certainly not try any of these additional measures unless you have learnt the appropriate details from a recognised and up-to-date local authority.

The spitting cobra deserves a special mention. As well as biting it can eject its poison fast and forcefully over several feet into the face and eyes of its victim. It is most important to wash the harmful material immediately from the eyes with copious amounts of water or of any other bland fluid available.

Other Venomous Animals

The many sorts of poisons, which many sorts of animals can inject into man, produce symptoms which, generally speaking, are similar to those from snake bite. As a first aider you will follow the principles of:

relieving pain with suitable tablets;
getting medical help rapidly;
resting the bitten part;
resting the patient in the Recovery Position (p. 112);
guarding him and his breathing if he vomits or collapses (p. 49);
giving Resuscitation if this is needed (p. 130).

Give first-aid treatment of inflamed skin by applying a bland, soothing preparation like *calamine lotion*, preferably in its oily form. The potent chemical histamine is a component of most of the poisons, so *antihistamine cream* smoothed into the skin can prove very useful. Unfortunately many people are sensitive to it; its use on them would worsen the inflammation. Apply this cream only on people whom you know to be unlikely to react badly to it.

Venomous Fish

The *sting ray's* sharp barb is found in its tail; as the tail lashes the barb bends up and can pierce a paddler's skin.

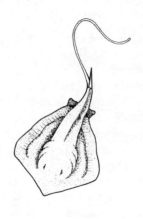

The *Weever fish* is yellow to brown and can be trodden on as it lies half-buried in sand, or it can hurt, if handled by trawlermen. One long poisonous spine lies by its gill cover but the parts, which generally pierce the unguarded foot or hand, are the half-a-dozen spines in the back.

The venom of both these fish is destroyed by heat. Relieve the pain as soon as possible by immersing the stung part, for at least half an hour, in water as hot as the patient can bear it, without being scalded. Look for any spines still in the skin and pull them out.

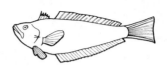

Jellyfish

Their tentacles carry stinging capsules, which discharge venom, leaving a row of weals on the attacked skin.

Flush the area with sea water to remove any poison on the surface.

(Do not use fresh water for this could stimulate activity of any undischarged capsules.)

Detach adhering tentacles gently and carefully using a towel or gloved hand after applying vinegar. (Do not try alcohol; this could activate more capsules to sting.) If there are no other means available, cover the tentacles with wet sand, which you then scrape off with a thin hard edge, like the back of a knife. Now wash the part with sea water.

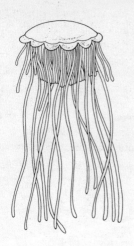

Insect Stings

Remove the sting if it is still present. A bee sting is barbed and tends to remain stuck in the human skin. It gets torn off the insect (who consequently will die). Stuck in the skin, it continues to pump out any venom it still holds. You should make any attempt to pull it out with fine forceps by grasping it as close to the skin as possible, to avoid squeezing more venom down. It is however better to try to scrape out the sting with a finger nail, as quickly as possible.

You can relieve pain with tablets or by applying a cold compress (p. 62). Do *not* apply things like ammonia or vinegar to the sting; their use has been discredited.

There are three potentially dangerous situations with insect stings when you must get medical help, or send the patient to hospital as rapidly as you can.

1. Stings in the mouth

The loose tissues in the mouth and at the back of the throat can react by swelling considerably, blocking up the airway and making breathing difficult. Get the patient to suck ice cubes; an iced 'lolly' will serve if nothing else is available.

2. Multiple stings

Many stings from a swarm of bees or wasps are threatening because of the large amount of venom injected.

3. Collapse after stinging

A state of collapse could follow stinging if the patient has an abnormally high sensitivity to the venom. The sensitivity can develop insidiously in someone who has considered himself immune. Rarely the insect sting can enter a blood vessel, giving a full concentration of venom to the blood stream. Treat the patient as for shock (p. 105) and rapidly obtain medical care. If he is a beekeeper ask if he has any medication, like anti-histamine tablets, prescribed for just such an emergency.

Ticks

Quite apart from their distressingly tenacious hold on the skin, some ticks can transmit diseases through their bite. They are about 5 mm long, flat, black or brown, and have four pairs of legs.

Do not try to pull or rub them off for this could leave some mouth-part in the wound. Clog their breathing by covering them with a heavy fluid, which could be liquid paraffin, machine or even salad oil. It may take half-an-hour for this to be effective. Then, if the tick has not fallen off, use forceps to remove it carefully, without squeezing.

You can also detach ticks by touching them with a lighted cigarette, but as ticks are so small you risk injuring the patient's skin.

Leeches

They do not poison but they stick to the skin to suck in blood. The bite itself is not painful. Do not try to pull them off for this could leave mouth-parts still embedded. They will let go if touched with a strong salt solution, alcohol or a mild acid like vinegar.

As their saliva contains substances which prevent blood clotting, the wounds may bleed for a long time after; use firmly-bandaged dressings to control this.

Leech bites frequently become infected; it would be wise to seek medical advice.

Plants

Some plants like nettles, or the giant hogweed, will sting and irritate. Cold water on the skin will help at once. After drying follow this by smoothing on calamine lotion or cream.

Remember that thorns of roses and other plants have been known to carry tetanus as they prick (see p. 9).

Some plants, like the cactus, can embed very many fine spines on a hand that has carelessly brushed against or grasped them. Press a piece of elastic adhesive bandage or Scotch tape over the area and then pull it off; it will bring the spines with it.

Questions

1. You do not give any medicines or tablets as part of your first-aid treatment. Yet this chapter mentions two cases where this rule should be broken. What are they?

2. A paddler limps in from a beach at low tide, with intense pain in one foot. He thinks he walked on something alive. What do you think happened? Can you do anything to help?

3. An experienced beekeeper deals with a swarming colony and is stung in a dozen places. He is confident that he needs no attention. A few minutes later he begins to sweat and feel very faint. What do you do?

4. At a picnic on the moors your elderly aunt cries out that she pricked her finger on putting her hand into a low bush. Two small painful spots on her finger are about 1 cm apart. Describe in detail what you should do.

17
Heat and Cold

Body Temperature

Many animals have a body temperature, which moves up and down to match, or be just a little above, the atmospheric temperatures in which they live. Human beings and other mammals share with birds the fact that their temperature is, or strives to be, more or less constant.

The average temperature of the healthy man is 37° Centigrade (or 98.6° Fahrenheit). It varies slightly according to whether he is very active or at rest. It is also a little higher in the evenings than in the early hours of the morning. So there are normal fluctuations of, perhaps, 1°C either way, and these are of no importance. The chemical processes, which govern life, will work well within that temperature range. A body temperature, which moves down below 36° C (96.8° F), progressively slows down the chemical reactions and thereby the actions and also the thinking power of the cold person. A move in the opposite direction, with body temperatures increasing beyond 38° C (100.4° F), can destroy many of the essential body chemicals concerned.

Specialised controlling centres in the brain receive messages about heat and cold from outpost informers like nerve endings in the skin. Acting on these the centres try to stabilise body temperature by sending, through other nerves, appropriate impulses to muscles, blood vessels, and sweat glands.

How Does the Body Keep Warm?

The living activity of tissue cells, their taking up of nourishment and converting it to biological energy, is the principal way heat develops in the body. This can be thought of as similar to (but much more complicated than) the heat produced during test-tube reactions in the chemistry laboratory.

If there is a captain of the body's heat production, it would undoubtedly be the liver. This large and busy organ has several hundred biochemical functions and is the warmest place in the body.

Muscle action is another heat producer. In cold weather man is uncomfortable if he keeps still. The sufferer tries to make himself warmer by being active and by moving limbs energetically. The body does this unasked by shivering; a great deal of heat can be engendered by this fast automatic muscle tremor of the chilled person.

To counter heat loss from the body surface, we wear clothing that traps insulating layers of air around the skin. The skin also plays an active part by becoming pale. Pallor in this case is due to reflex narrowing of the blood vessels under the skin. This reduces the volume of warm blood coursing just below the body surfaces and therefore the heat that can be lost to the outside. The blood volume, which has been 'squeezed' out of these skin vessels, now augments that in the depths of the body. This concept of the cold protective outer 'shell' and of the inner warm 'core' has already been described in the chapter on shock (p. 102). The richer supply of blood in the 'core' is serving the deeper body organs that maintain life.

How Does the Body Keep Cool?

What of the person who is troubled by an overheated atmosphere or by the fever of an illness? How does the body try to keep its temperature normal?

Here again the skin plays a major role. Initially it reddens as its vessels automatically widen and become engorged with heat-bearing blood. Much of the heat dissipates from the skin's surface into the surrounding air.

The next process is that of perspiration. Watery fluid pours out of sweat glands to coat the skin. It now evaporates into the air. We are accustomed to the way in which water can evaporate; we see it every time the water level gradually lowers in a dish left out in the sun or when we boil a saucepan of water. This physical change from a fluid to a vapour state is not simple; it demands a great deal of heat. The water in the saucepan does not turn to vapour as soon as it reaches boiling point: the saucepan will need to remain over the flame or electric ring, taking in much more heat, before vapour is seen to rise from the water surface. Sweating by itself is not enough to reduce someone's temperature; the really effective event is the *evaporation* of sweat into the air, using up heat, which it takes away from the body.

This mechanism is not without its disadvantages. It works well when the sweating person is in a dry atmosphere. But if he is in a very humid atmosphere the air is less ready to accept more water vapour, and evaporation from the skin surface is slowed down.

Another, and very important, point is that sweat does not consist of water only. It carries with it a certain amount of salty chemicals taken from the body. Anyone who has sweat running down his face on to his mouth can testify to the strong, salty taste experienced if he runs his tongue over his lips. In moderate quantities this salt loss is not damaging, but if sweating is very heavy the salty concentration, which forms on the skin surface, interferes with easy evaporation of water. Also, and more harmfully, the inside of the body can become significantly depleted of salts, which are essential to its well-being.

Measuring the Temperature

Use a clinical thermometer, which is made of glass and therefore must be handled carefully. Hold it by the upper end and not by the mercury reservoir at the lower end. Otherwise the heat of your finger may give incorrect results.

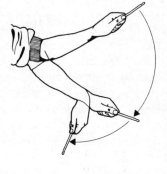

First wash it in cold water and dry it gently. Now you must shake down the mercury column which may be up in the narrow channel of the ther-mometer body. This is quite easy:

(a) Grasp the thermometer firmly at the top.

(b) Give yourself a clear space so that you do not hit the thermometer against anything and break it.

(c) Bend your arm up at the elbow and then rapidly straighten it down.

(d) Immediately follow this through with a sharp flick to bend the hand at the wrist.

You may have to shake several times to get the mercury fully down.

Put the thermometer gently under the patient's tongue. Ask him to close his lips on it, but not to bite. Keep the thermometer there for two minutes (supporting it outside with your fingers if necessary). During this time the patient should not try to speak. Some thermometers claim to give a reading in half-a-minute, but all too often that is unreliably optimistic.

Reading the result may prove difficult if the mercury line is very

thin. Hold the thermometer at eye
level and slowly rotate it until at one
point (sometimes quite suddenly) you
see the mercury. Its upper level will
show the reading against the temperature scale engraved on the glass.
Now wash and dry the thermometer
and put it away safely.

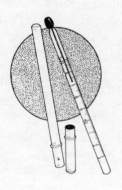

If the patient cannot close his
mouth, is not fully co-operative, is a
small child, or is unconscious, you
should not use his mouth, but his
armpit. Dry the armpit area, tuck the
thermometer there and hold the arm
close against it for four minutes.
Armpit temperatures generally are
½° C (1° F) below mouth temperatures.

Heat Exhaustion and Heat Stroke

The word 'sunstroke' is little used now. It had covered various ill-
defined troubles from heat and proved too vague, especially as the
sunshine itself was not the responsible factor.

Harmful effects of excessive heat have been classified into two
groups, *Heat Exhaustion* where there has been much sweating and
Heat Stroke where sweating has been impaired or absent. Since it is
useful to compare the two, point by point, they are set out in tabular
form.

The general health of the patient can greatly affect his response to
heat. Heart and chest troubles make him much more susceptible. Also
please remember that elderly people, babies, and small children are far
more likely to collapse in overheated states.

Heat Exhaustion	Heat Stroke
The circumstances are likely to be those of someone who has been active for hours or even days in very hot conditions.	*The circumstances* would be those of extreme heat in a very humid atmosphere, for example, someone in a tropical area, marshy on the ground and with many trees forming a canopy of leaves overhead. Between ground and leaves there is a hot mass of air saturated with moisture. Absence of wind or breeze worsens the situation.
As he becomes warmer he perspires heavily. Sweat constantly forms on his skin; its evaporation tends to keep him cool.	
By perspiring he has been losing a great deal of fluid. He has also lost much of his body salts, as they accompany the sweat.	The patient begins to perspire but sweat cannot evaporate from him into an air already heavily, fully, charged with water vapour. He cannot lose heat; his temperature rises steeply. Soon the brain's temperature-regulating mechanism breaks down and sweating ceases.
	Any excessively high and fast rise of temperature may cause such a breakdown, even in a dry and temperate atmosphere. Therefore another possible cause of heat-stroke could be the rapidly raised fever of some infections. This includes certain phases of malaria.
The symptoms are thirst, tiredness, restlessness. The patient also may have a headache and feel sick and dizzy.	*The symptoms* at first are similar to those of heat exhaustion but more intense and likely to develop faster. The patient will have weakness, dizziness, nausea, vomiting, and headache.
Depleted of salts his muscles may react by going into strong contractions. Therefore another likely feature is the onset of cramps, and these can be severe—especially in the legs or abdomen.	He will feel very hot.
	Since he has not sweated much, he has not lost much salt; therefore cramps will not be a feature.

Heat Exhaustion	Heat Stroke
Eventually the patient could faint or collapse.	In severe cases the patient may be delirious or have convulsions and rapidly become unconscious.
When you examine him you find features very similar to those of shock. His skin is pale and moist, with cheeks appearing sunken; pulse and breathing are fast and feeble. Because of the protective action of sweat evaporation his temperature is likely to be normal or only slightly raised.	*When you examine him* you find his skin quite dry, very red, and very hot. His pulse is fast and forceful and so is his breathing. His temperature will be high, in the region of 41° C (106° F) or more.
Treatment is simple. Get the patient out of the heat into a cool shelter, loosen his clothes and put him at rest. If his consciousness is clouded let him be in the Recovery Position (p. 112).	*Treatment* is directed to cooling as fast as possible since very high temperatures can be fatal. Move the patient to a cool shelter, remove his clothing and put him in the Recovery Position (p. 112).
Dry his skin with a towel.	Fan him with large cloths or sheets of paper, or use an electric fan. Sponge the trunk and limbs with cold water. Or wrap him in a sheet soaked in water; as it warms up keep on renewing the water. A cold compress (p. 62) on the forehead will also help.
If he is conscious and able to swallow give drinks to replace what he has lost (see p. 175). Let him take this slowly in sips, for fast gulps might induce vomiting. Let him take *at least* two, full tumblers. The drink can be cold water or fruit juice; add a quarter of a teaspoonful of ordinary salt to each tumbler.	Do not however use ice-cold water, nor try to bring the temperature right down to normal. Aim for no lower than 38°–39° C (101°–102° F) Once this has been achieved cover the patient lightly with a dry sheet.
The patient is likely to recover well in a relatively short time. But it is wise to get medical advice, and essential to do so if he is unconscious.	Watch him and keep checking the temperature every five or ten minutes. If it rises resume the cooling measure.
	You must get medical help or an ambulance as soon as possible.

Frostbite

A part exposed to intense cold becomes severely affected in two ways. First the blood vessels of the area constrict, so that the skin loses its pink colour and becomes blue or very white. Second there can be freezing and disruption of the tissues by the formation of minute ice crystals within them. Gangrene could develop in very severe cases.

The areas most likely to be affected are exposed parts and extremities of the body, like the nose, ears, chin, fingers, and toes. Frostbite begins with tingling, numbness and paling of the skin. These warnings should be taken seriously before the condition worsens. Deprived of a proper blood supply, which could come to its rescue, frostbitten skin is in a very weakened state. It has to be handled with great gentleness. This forbids you to try to reinvigorate it by massage; old ideas like rubbing with snow are dangerous and must be discarded.

Bring the patient indoors as soon as possible. He is allowed to walk short distances on frostbitten feet. But once the feet have thawed after being frostbitten the skin temporarily cannot cope with the pressure of walking; carry the patient or transport him by stretcher.

The patient is still outdoors

Remove any potentially constricting object, like a ring or garter, which could further impede circulation.

Cover the frostbitten area generously with something warm and dry. The patient can cup an unaffected hand over nose, chin or ear; he can tuck frostbitten fingers, under his clothes, into his armpit.

The patient has been brought indoors

1. Get him into a warm room and, if his clothes are frozen, replace them by warm coverings.

2. Rewarm the frostbitten part. This will be done gradually by exposure to warm air. Where it is practicable, this can be done fast by immersing in a container of water at 42° C (108° F). In the absence of a thermometer you can judge this temperature as one that is just comfortable to bear by an elbow dipped in the water. Discontinue this immersion in warm water after half-an-hour or earlier if the limb has regained its colour, feeling, and pliability. Maintain the temperature by adding hot water to the container, but be careful not to pour it

directly over the limb and use your hand to mix it thoroughly. If a glove or shoe is frozen on to the frostbitten part, immerse it with the limb in the warm water before attempting to remove it. You must *not* try to warm the part by using a fire or a hot-water bottle.

3. Dry the frostbitten skin by dabbing it gently with cotton wool or a suitable cloth. Do not rub; the skin would not stand it.

4. Now keep it loosely covered with a dry cloth.

5. Elevate a limb, which has been affected at its extremity. This will reduce pain and swelling.

6. Get medical advice or have the patient taken to hospital. Do not let him walk on a foot, which has just been thawed out. If it is quite unavoidable that he should walk, he should do this before the foot is rewarmed.

Hypothermia

Basically the word 'hypothermia' means little more than a temperature below normal. However, medically, it is used for situations in which the patient's core (deep body) temperature becomes so low that vital functions are dangerously reduced.

The hypothermic patient is by medical definition, one whose body core temperature is below 35° C (95° F). You cannot measure such temperatures with the ordinary clinical thermometer; doctors use a special low-reading thermometer which will register down to 25° C (77° F). The ways the patient and his body are affected by such severe chilling is shown in the diagram opposite. It is only a general description as so much depends on the patient's general health before cooling and on his age. Brain and heart are the main sufferers; their biochemical processes slow down and eventually stop as the temperature decreases.

Hypothermia can happen in many ways and is by no means restricted to arctic conditions, mountain heights, ocean exposures or winter severities. It is a general threat where warmth cannot be adequately maintained by suitable shelter, heating, clothing, and covering.

There are several ways in which hypothermia could occur e.g. to the sailor at sea or the baby in his cot,

Exposure: The Hill Climber

In the valley, where it is warm and sunny, a young man joins an organised walking trek to the hills. He has dressed fairly lightly and is surprised to see how much his companions are wearing.

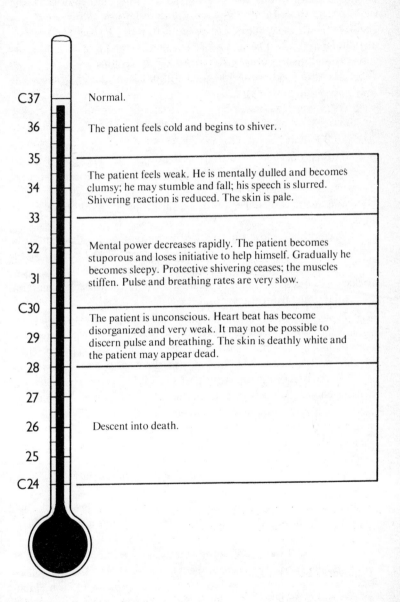

C37 — Normal.

36 — The patient feels cold and begins to shiver.

35

34 — The patient feels weak. He is mentally dulled and becomes clumsy; he may stumble and fall; his speech is slurred. Shivering reaction is reduced. The skin is pale.

33

32 — Mental power decreases rapidly. The patient becomes stuporous and loses initiative to help himself. Gradually he becomes sleepy. Protective shivering ceases; the muscles

31 — stiffen. Pulse and breathing rates are very slow.

C30 — The patient is unconscious. Heart beat has become disorganized and very weak. It may not be possible to discern pulse and breathing. The skin is deathly white and

29 — the patient may appear dead.

28

27

26 — Descent into death.

25

C24

As the party ascends he is energetic and he sweats, the moisture being retained in his clothes. Soon clouds cover the sun and, up in the heights, strong winds are playing. His damp clothes add to the coldness he feels. Feeling abnormally tired he slows down and falls behind the others. Walking becomes an effort and he becomes clumsy, stumbling at times. The group leader hails him but his mind has lost its usual friendliness and he gives irrational, querulous replies.

After struggling for another hour he falls down and is both mentally and physically too weak to rise.

Treatment

1. This should have started with prevention, the group leader recognising the inadequacy of the man's clothing and ensuring proper covering before they set out.

2. When the walker began to lag, this, too, he should have noted, making him stop and rest.

3. Preferably a closed hut should be sought but, if this cannot be quickly reached, treatment continues in the open. The best available shelter from the wind should be used, finding protection by trees or rocks. The cold man would be made to sit or lie on protective material to insulate him from the ground.

4. From the party, spare, dry clothing could be found to replace the cold, wet ones. If the moist clothes could not be removed, then at least they would be covered by others. Plastic bags or sheets are excellent insulators. How to use blankets is described on p. 185.

5. At the first opportunity the patient should have warm, sweetened drinks: cocoa would be ideal. In the absence of fluids he could eat sugar, glucose or chocolate. But alcohol is never given; by dilating the skin's blood vessels it would increase the loss of heat from the body surface and also draw away blood from the heart and brain in the body 'core'.

6. The leader now uses the fittest members of the party to send for help.

7. During the wait the leader's attitude matters greatly: he will express cheerful expectancy to maintain the patient's morale.

Once a walker has collapsed the matter has become very urgent. He is a stretcher case. He is given drinks only if still conscious and co-operative. Warming is essential and could be done by other members of the party huddling around him, or by someone sharing a wide sleeping bag with him.

Immersion: The Seaman

Wearing a lifebelt over ordinary clothing and coat, a seaman falls overboard into a very cold sea. By the time he is rescued he is motionless, with blanched skin and seems to be dead.

Treatment

1. The seaman began his own treatment by avoiding movement while waiting to be picked up. He did just enough to 'curl up' with legs and arms folded over the trunk and chest and to keep his head above water and no more.

Swimming and splashing in the cold sea would have allowed the skin to dissipate heat more quickly from his body. Water extracts heat from any object in it far more than would air at the same temperature.

2. You must try Resuscitation (p. 130) at once to the unbreathing and apparently dead. The very cold state of their bodies may make it almost impossible to detect any minimal heart and breathing action still present. A medical aphorism states that 'victims of severe hypothermia are never dead until they are warm and dead'.

In these conditions of intense cooling there is a slight risk that chest compression might turn the weakened, but still useful, beats into ineffectual heart muscle tremors which cannot pump blood. But if these beats cannot be detected after one minute's careful testing, there is no other possible decision than to start Artificial Ventilation and Chest Compression.

Because the beat of a very cold heart is so slow the rate of chest compression should begin at 30 to 40 a minute, that is half the ordinary rate.

3. This deeply hypothermic patient needs rapid rewarming, once resuscitation has succeeded or is not needed. If possible he is put into a bath at 42° C (108° F)—even if he is unconscious. The temperature can be judged as that just bearable by the elbow dipped into the water.

It is wise to immerse the patient's trunk in the warm water but, as far as can be done, to leave the arms and legs out of the water. This apparent paradox is due to the fact that the large blood vessels of the limbs react quicker to the new warmth than do the vessels of the trunk. As they widen rapidly the flow in them picks up and passes their colder blood into the circulation of the body core. This will cause a temporary but marked further drop of body core temperature. The 'after-drop', as it is called, can be reduced by rewarming the trunk first.

Once the patient has a satisfactory pulse and respiration and is normally conscious get him out of the bath and wrap him up warmly.

4. When he is conscious and can swallow, give the patient warm sweet drinks.

5. Medical help or hospital admission is urgently needed.

Domestic Hypothermia

In the armchair of his living room an old man has dozed off. A very sharp frost supervenes and the cold gradually overcomes him as he sleeps.

He is more susceptible than most. Trying to economise he had no fire. At his age blood circulation is impaired and some glands which stoke up body energy are poorly active. Also tranquilisers and sedatives, which he is taking, have a temperature-lowering effect.

Next morning he is still in the chair, almost unrousable. He barely talks and is not easy to understand. White and puffy, his skin is very cold to touch even where it is well covered by clothes. His pulse and breathing are slow and weak.

In the nursery of the house next door a much-loved and well-cared-for baby has been very quiet overnight. The morning shows that coverings had slipped from his cot.

Like the elderly, babies are easy victims of cold. They have a relatively thin layer of heat-insulating fat. Their body surface area, from which heat can be lost, is relatively large in comparison with the body volume. In the baby and small child the brain's temperature controlling nerve centres are not yet fully developed. Babies do not have the rewarming help of shivering, and in sleep they lie still instead of moving a little as do adults.

The hypothermic baby will show features similar to those of the hypothermic adult. In some cases however, the baby's skin can be not white but deceptively rosy pink.

Treatment

This patient's temperature is not as low as that of the seaman who was, so suddenly and rapidly, chilled in the sea. The domestic slow cooling had been accompanied by gradual chemical changes in the body. The return to normal needs to be an equally gradual readjustment. Fast warming would rush the heart into forcible action for which it is not yet ready: the patient would die of heart failure. It would be similar to stalling an old car engine by trying to change it from ticking over in neutral gear to shooting forward in top gear.

1. *Put the patient in the Recovery Position* (p. 112) in bed.
2. *Cover him fully* but loosely with blankets.

3. *Heat the room* to 28°–30° C (82°–86° F) and let the patient warm up slowly. Do *not* heat him or his bed directly with such things as hot-water bottles or electric blankets.

4. *Give warm, sweetened drinks* like cocoa (or whatever is suitable for the baby's age) if the patient is conscious and co-operative (see pp. 115, 220). Never give alcohol.

5. *Get medical help or ambulance.* This is particularly important when the patient is unconscious or is a baby; urgent hospital care is probably needed.

There is one other primary treatment instruction; *suspect the possibility of hypothermia* especially in the aged and the very young. Too many victims have been found in their beds by well-meaning people who thought that they were just having a bit of extra sleep, and left them to sink into further depths of body cold.

The Chilled Patient: Treatment Summary

1. Resuscitate if necessary.
2. Rewarm. As a generalization:

if cooling has been fast: rewarm fast.
if cooling has been slow: rewarm slowly.

3. Dry, if necessary, and cover.
4. Put in the Recovery Position.
5. Seek medical help.

Covering Someone Warmly

Retaining the patient's own warmth is a very important part of many first-aid treatments. In an emergency you can improvise covering from over-coats, large towels or sacks.

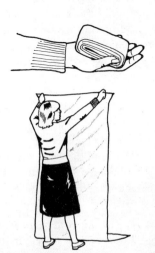

The planned first-aid kit can include plastic sheets, which are excellent heat insulators, light in weight and easy to pack. Also the *Rescue Blanket* made of thin, but strong, metal foil can fit in a pocket but will unfold to a good size for covering and wrapping round a patient.

In very cold circumstances remember that one-sixth of the body's heat loss can happen at the head area, which therefore you must keep covered.

Always aim to keep the warm coverings loosely applied, even when you tuck them in.

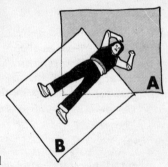

Two blanket covering

Two large blankets can be manoeuvred into a most efficient protection against the cold.

1. Place Blanket A on the ground and Blanket B diagonally across one of its corner areas. If necessary you can lay a plastic sheet over Blanket B to help, even further, to retain heat. Get the patient lying on Blanket B so that his feet are a little way from its lower edge and his armpits are at its upper edge. Have his shoulders, head and raised arms lie on Blanket A.

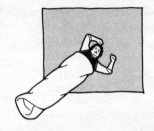

2. Turn the bottom of Blanket B over the patient's feet, and then tuck each side of the blanket round the trunk and legs.

3. Fold the upper part of Blanket A over and down to form a line near the patient's head.

4. Bring one 'wing' of Blanket A over the patient's trunk and tuck it in Let one fold come close against the side of the head and curve over the scalp.

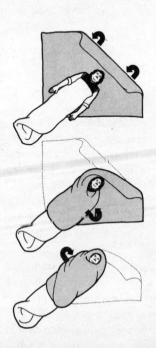

5. Bring the second 'wing' of Blanket A round the other side of the face and chin, across the trunk and tuck it in under the opposite side.

The patient is now fully covered, except for his face.

Questions

1. Why could it be said that hypothermia at home is especially likely to concern the two extremes of age?

2. One very cold winter morning the staff of a small factory arrive to find a power failure; no lights or machinery will work. The night watchman does not report and is found unrousably asleep in his office. The manager talks of dismissing him. Describe your advice and actions.

3. Detail the way you take the temperature of (1) a compliant adult and (2) an agitated child.

4. As you try to dig out your car from a snowbank a quarter of a mile from home the fingers of one hand become frostbitten. What do you do?

5. Explain the value to the body of (1) skin redness, (2) skin pallor, (3) shivering, and (4) sweating under different circumstances of extreme heat and cold.

6. Your companion on a canal barge has been at the tiller for a long time in a cold wind and fine rain. After he has made some steering errors you suggest taking over. He refuses angrily. Are you facing a social, medical or a navigational problem? How do you act?

7. Your neighbour has used a weekend of brilliant sunshine to dig his garden unremittingly. Then you see him pale and collapsed in a deck chair. How could you help and why?

18
Some Medical Conditions

Asthma

In a serious asthmatic attack three things are happening to the air tubes (A) of the patient's lungs. The tubes tense and constrict so that the passage for air (C) becomes smaller. The lining of the tubes (B) becomes much thicker than normal making the passage yet smaller. The situation worsens as this swollen lining secretes thick mucus into the remaining space. With these partly blocked tubes the patient is wheezing, having great difficulty getting air in and out of his lungs.

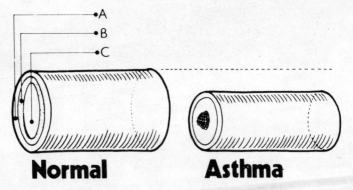

Normal **Asthma**

In the asthma-prone patient three likely things can set this off: allergy, infection, and emotion. In whatever way the attack may have begun the emotional factor can worsen it. Discomfort and anxiety builds up in the victim who finds his breathing progressively more obstructed. Severe attacks can last a few minutes or extend to several hours.

Your first-aid contribution will be to get the patient to relax physically and mentally and to position him to help the mechanics of breathing. Be calm and give clear advice, engendering an atmosphere of confidence.

1. In a severe attack call a doctor.
2. Let in fresh (not cold) air.
3. If the patient has any tablets or inhalers for the emergency see that he uses them. But beware of overdoses and check that he has not already exceeded the dosage which a doctor had prescribed.

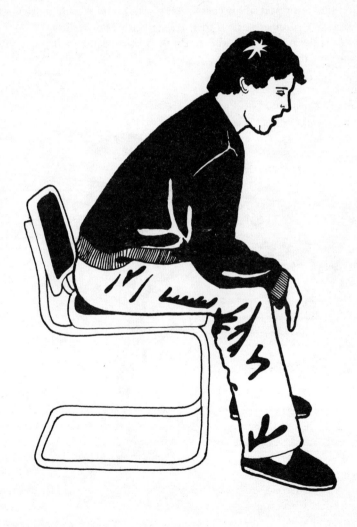

4. Do not let the patient crouch forwards. Whether he is standing or sitting he should hold his back straight, as this helps the work of the chest muscles. But he may lean forwards on a comfortable support if he wishes. Beware of feather-filled pillows as some asthmatics are allergic to feathers.

5. Ask him to relax all other parts of the body (limbs, neck, face). This can play a part in reducing the tension in his air tubes.

6. Advise him to concentrate breathing movements at waist level and the lower part of his chest. Many patients, with asthma, struggle to move the upper part of their chests, with poor results.

7. If the patient feels able to drink, a warm drink of strong coffee can sometimes help him.

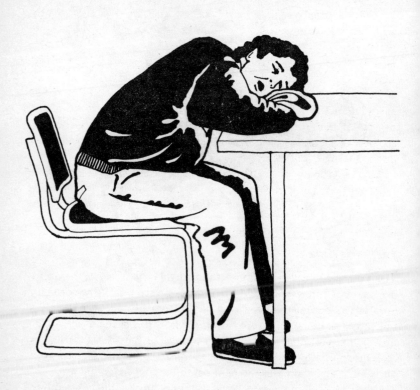

Heart Attack

A muscle working actively needs, and usually receives, a more plentiful blood supply than when it is at rest. Were the blood flow to it restricted, the muscle reacts by producing pain.

The muscles that form the beating walls of the heart get their blood from vessels called the *coronary arteries*. As the heart is constantly in action it is important that these arteries allow an unimpeded blood flow.

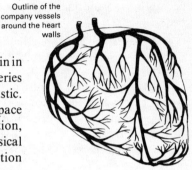

Outline of the company vessels around the heart walls

Angina

This is the name given to chest pain in someone whose coronary arteries have become narrow and inelastic. The blood supply cannot keep pace with the need of the heart in exertion, when the patient does some physical effort or is subject to strong emotion like excitement or anxiety.

Pain is felt behind the breastbone and, by nerve connections, it may spread up to the throat, jaw, and shoulders or down the arm, especially on the left side. It may be accompanied by breathlessness. Generally, as soon as the patient becomes quiet again and his heart beat slows down, the pain will clear.

If you find someone in anginal pain help him to sit down, loosen any tight clothing, and let him keep his back upright, which helps breathing. If he has any tablets prescribed for anginal attacks, ask him to use them.

The Heart Attack

The true heart attack is more than angina. It is called *coronary occlusion* or *coronary thrombosis* indicating that one of the coronary arteries has become blocked by a blood clot (thrombosis). Here it is not just a matter of a reduced flow; the flow has been cut off by the obstructing clot. The area of heart muscle served by that artery is receiving practically no blood at all. The heart cannot rest; it tries to go on beating and therefore the pain continues and increases.

This pain is felt in the same areas as that of angina, but it is far more intense, with a very tight, gripping sensation in the chest. The patient is shocked. He is pale and breathless; he may be sweating. His pulse is fast and weak; it may be irregular. The condition is serious and it may be fatal.

The patient's distress and fear can unfortunately worsen the situation as emotion itself may now activate a heart which should be allowed to beat as peacefully as is possible under the circumstances. Your psychological approach is as important as your physical help.

1. Get the patient to rest at once. Treat him where he is found. If a bed or couch is present get him on it, but do not expend time or the patient's energy by moving him to a distant bed.

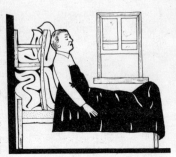

2. Loosen tight clothes.

3. Keep the patient warm by loose covering, and allow fresh air.

4. If his breathing is difficult he would be easier sitting upright. You can use a small chair overturned at the end of the bed and banked with pillows as a bed rest. Otherwise he should be lying down.

5. Send urgently for medical help, explaining the nature of the case.

6. Be sympathetic, showing that you realise the extent of his pain. At the same time be as comfortingly reassuring as you can, intimating that the attack will come under control. Avoid having 'helpers' crowding round and fussing. Do not let them try to give him brandy or a similar drink.

If the patient's breathing stops, begin resuscitation immediately (p. 130). However never try this while he is still breathing; you would only make matters dangerously worse.

Not all attacks of coronary thrombosis are accompanied by agonising pain. In a few cases symptoms are relatively mild, the patient may even believe that he is being troubled by nothing more than 'bad indigestion'. If you are at all uncertain about the nature of his pain act for safety. Put him at rest and get medical advice.

Acute Heart Failure

There is another type of heart attack, which is free of pain because its cause is not the blocking-off of the blood supply from a coronary artery. A weakened or infirm heart muscle may suddenly cease to act efficiently. It no longer pumps blood adequately from the heart chambers. The heart becomes overfilled with blood. This congestion spreads backwards along the veins from the lungs. The lungs in turn become congested, and cannot function properly.

The patient (sometimes waking from sleep) is distressingly breathless. His breathing sounds wet and bubbly (not sharply wheezy as in asthma). Sometimes he is coughing up watery sputum, which may be blood-tinged. He is pale or blue.

Treat this exactly as you would the coronary thrombosis. In this case you must have him sitting up rather than lying down, to facilitate his chest's breathing movements. Get medical help urgently.

Stroke

Stroke or 'apoplexy' is a mishap to a blood vessel in some part of the brain. It can be a clot blocking an artery, so depriving some brain tissue of its blood supply. It can be the rupture of a vessel, with bleeding.

The consequences depend on how rapidly these happen and on the area of the brain concerned. Commonly it causes loss of power or feeling in an arm or leg (or both) on one side of the body. Sometimes other functions are affected: sight may be dimmed, speech may become slurred; memory may be weakened or the patient's ability to select correct words from his vocabulary may be lost.

The attack could happen very suddenly with falling or with unconsciousness. Or a stroke may begin quite mildly by finding a hand or foot numb and clumsy, and having difficulty in walking or grasping. A patient may wake in the morning with these handicaps after having gone to bed normally the previous night. The condition may worsen over the next few hours.

One of your roles as first aider is to suspect the likelihood of a stroke when only minor symptoms occur. Since one cannot know at the onset how an attack will progress, or whether unconsciousness will supervene, put the patient in the Recovery Position (p. 112). Loosen his clothing and cover him warmly. If possible have him in bed. Send for medical help and keep a close watch on the patient: you may have to help him if he vomits or becomes incontinent.

Remember that the apparently helpless, mindless patient, who cannot properly express himself, may yet be perceiving and thinking normally. Guard your speech. Show him all the reassurance and sympathy you can.

Epilepsy

This disorder of brain action gives attacks of temporarily-impaired consciousness. Sometimes epilepsy arises for no clear reason; sometimes it is related to a recognisable physical cause such as brain illnesses or damage left after head injuries.

A minor and a major form exist.

Minor attacks

In the minor form (known by the French words 'Petit Mal') the patient quite suddenly stops whatever he is doing. He 'goes blank' for a few seconds, but he does not necessarily fall. When he comes to, he may carry on normally and the briefness of the attack may make it barely noticeable. Or the patient may move about vaguely and you should then keep quietly by his side to prevent his coming to harm.

Major attacks

The major form ('Grand Mal') brings about falls, unconsciousness, and jerking fits. These attacks vary very much from epileptic to epileptic. The events and the times described below can give only an average picture.

	The Events	**First-Aid Action**
Patient Conscious	Just before the attack most patients have no hint of its imminence. A few patients may briefly get their own style of warning such as dimness of vision, noises in the ears, feeling faint or illusions of peculiar smells or tastes. Some move about with purposeless activity.	If warning features do present themselves, these could allow the patient to lie down before the fall.
Patient Unconscious	Quite suddenly the patient falls, silent, and unconscious. Sometimes a patient may give one cry.	Bear in mind that he might have injured himself in the fall.
	The fit now proceeds in three stages. 1. (Lasts half to one minute.) With muscles rigid the patient lies quite still, not breathing properly. He may become blue in the face.	Guard his airway (p. 36) Loosen tight clothing at his neck and waist.

2. (Lasts 30 to 45 seconds.) Jerking begins and can build up vigorously, affecting the limbs and the whole body. In these uncontrolled muscle movements the patient could bite his tongue (with blood showing at the mouth), and he could be incontinent of urine. He may froth at the mouth. Breathing remains poor and could be harsh and noisy.

Do not try to restrain the jerking: let it happen. If limbs are knocking against a moveable piece of furniture shift it. If it cannot be moved quickly push a buffering pad (cushion, rolled-up coat) between it and the limbs. Do not try to put anything between the teeth to protect the tongue for this may require harmfully forcing the jaws apart. Mop away froth to prevent its inhalation when the patient breathes in.

---

3. (Lasts a few minutes, but rarely this can extend into hours.) The patient stops jerking and lies relaxed. His breathing and colour return to normal.

Give the general attention for unconsciousness (p. 110) with special attention to keeping his airway clear and to checking for any injuries. Place him in the Recovery Position (p. 112) unless injuries preclude this.

Patient Conscious

He recovers consciousness. He may be alert and normal or he may be vague and confused for some time. Many feel sleepy.

Watch him closely until he has returned to his normal mind. Let him rest if all is now well and you know that the patient is accustomed to attacks, and that he can look after himself or be looked after by his family: do not send him to hospital. But, if he is injured, or is a stranger or if he has had no previous epileptic attacks, you should call a doctor or send him to hospital by ambulance.

The epileptic state

Most epileptics, helped by modern treatment, have attacks infrequently. Rarely however the patient may, on the same day, have a succession of attacks at short, and decreasing, intervals. In this dangerous situation you should get medical help at once.

Hysteria

Men are as prone to hysteria as are women. The hysterical patient is an anxious and frightened person but not a malingerer. Frustration at work, in life's opportunities, in finance or in family life can be typical factors. The hysteric acts unconsciously on a concept that people are more sympathetic to physical ills than to psychological ones. He or she presents a 'cry for help' in the form of symptoms like pain, faintness, shaking or loss of power. Thereby a diagnosis of hysteria is difficult. It could be dangerous if mistakenly a true physical condition is disregarded. When, as could well happen, you are uncertain give the physical possibility the benefit of the doubt with appropriate first aid.

A strong clue to hysteria is the way the patients may grossly exaggerate symptoms, occasionally to the point of absurdity. For instance, while breathing powerfully, they may exclaim that breathing is impossible. Or they could agitate a limb which they believe to be paralysed. They may be noisily shouting or crying.

They may collapse, silent and motionless, as if unconscious. But, on careful handling, you find the muscles to be in good tone; if you lift an arm slightly and then let it go it stays up or descends slowly instead of falling limply. They may half open and move their eyes to assess what is going on.

Treatment

Do not treat a hysteric as if he were to blame. The patient believes in the symptoms and is truly unhappy. Do not give slaps or throw water.

Get as many people off the scene as possible; a 'cry for help' will quieten down in the absence of an audience. Speak reassuringly and very firmly, rather than sympathetically, so that the patient accepts you to be in charge and realises that there is no imminent danger. You can calm with instructions like: 'Your breathing is getting better. Now sit up straight. Take deep breaths and let them out slowly. Relax the rest of your body.'

Do not use phrases like 'Pull yourself together', which are meaningless. Do not say 'There is nothing the matter with you' for this will not be believed and your helpful authority will be discredited. There certainly is something the matter, although not what the patient fears. He must consult the doctor later for full help in identifying and coping with the true cause.

Diabetes

Digestion turns starchy and sweet foods into glucose, and our blood always contains a certain amount of this type of sugar. The body uses it as material for building tissues, and as fuel for their energy. Also glucose is essential for the proper working of the brain and nervous system.

In health the amount of glucose in the blood is automatically controlled. It fluctuates between an upper and a lower level of normal, never rising or falling beyond these, and usually lying somewhere between the two (A).

GLUCOSE LEVELS IN BLOOD

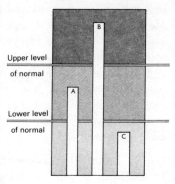

In the diabetic patient, however, the body's ability to use up glucose is faulty. Glucose accumulates and so the glucose load of the blood rises above the normal upper level (B). If this rise is very high the patient becomes unwell, unable to benefit properly from the starchy and sweet foods he eats. In long-standing and severe cases he loses weight and strength; he may become drowsy. He may even reach the point of passing into a coma. Generally this happens very gradually so that before the patient's ill health has reached this stage it becomes obvious that he is unwell and he has sought medical care.

Under treatment some diabetics receive tablets or self-administered injections that will bring about the action on glucose, which their bodies are no longer able to perform unaided. And that will correct the amount of glucose in the blood to the normal limits. But now the blood's glucose is no longer automatically regulated. It is dependent on the dose and time of medication, on the eating routine of patients, and on the amount of physical work they do.

If a treated patient expends little energy, if he eats too much or if he takes insufficient medication, the glucose will (temporarily at least) move to abnormally high levels again. However as soon as he resumes his proper routine this error will be corrected.

On the other hand the patient may give himself too big a dose of medication, do unusually heavy physical work (using up a great deal of glucose) or miss a meal. In that case the glucose level could descend below the lower level of normal (C). This gives very rapid deterioration in a few minutes, an emergency which may need immediate help from the first aider.

With this abnormally small amount of glucose in his blood the diabetic begins to feel hungry, faint, and perhaps cold. If he recognises what is happening to him and knows what to do he will quickly eat something sweet. Like many diabetics under treatment he may carry glucose tablets or sweets for such an emergency. Sometimes, however, his brain, affected by glucose deficiency, may not be working properly and he loses the initiative to help himself. He becomes pale, sweaty and tremulous, with a fast pulse. His co-ordination is poor so that he walks badly and his speech may be thick and difficult to understand. He may become irrational and aggressive. Unfortunately bystanders sometimes fail to understand his condition, judging him to be drunk. The patient may soon pass into a coma which could be fatal.

First-aid treatment

Suspect immediately a condition of low blood sugar. Suspicion may be confirmed if you are able to search the patient and find that he carries a card or a bracelet badge stating that he is diabetic, or if he has a syringe and medication (such as insulin for injection) or glucose tablets about him.

Act fast before the patient becomes unconscious and unable to swallow. Give him sugar in some form, preferably dissolved in water. Two or three tablets of glucose are ideal. If they are not available give lumps or teaspoonfuls of ordinary sugar; his body will quickly convert it to glucose. Chocolate, honey, jam, cake, biscuits or anything sweet, can be alternatives.

Should the patient have become aggressive, refusing to take what he is offered, your task is difficult. Sometimes casting a little granulated sugar into his open mouth may overcome this.

After receiving sweet material the patient is likely to return to his normal self in a very few minutes. It is then a good thing to give him a second sweet dose as a safety, maintenance, measure. Do not be afraid of giving him too much; excess sugar in his system is a temporary minor nuisance but insufficient sugar is an immediate danger.

If the patient has become unconscious do not try to give him anything by mouth. Place him in the Recovery Position (p. 112) and get medical help urgently.

Food Poisoning

This term is often used unjustifiably for any attack of diarrhoea and vomiting. It should be restricted to cases definitely due to bacterial infection of food. The bacteria may be alive in the food eaten; after a day or two of developing within the intestines they cause the illness. On the other hand bacteria may have produced poisons which remain quite unaffected by the heat of cooking—heat which kill the bacteria. Once swallowed the poisons give symptoms in a few hours.

First aid comes into the picture through a simple measure which can considerably relieve the patient's distress before he receives medical help. His feeling of wretchedness is due not only to bacterial poisons but also to the way copious vomit and loose stools make him lose fluid and certain salts.

He should replace these by suitable drinks. Advise him to take them as the pleasantly salty preparations used in commercial meat or yeast extracts. Alternatively he can have fresh orange or lemon juice with sugar and a pinch of salt. About a quarter of a teaspoonful of salt to each tumbler will be right.

He should take the drinks tepid if possible, and in slow sips. Hot or cold, or gulped fast the drinks could reflexly stimulate the bowel to increase diarrhoea and vomiting.

Fluid replacement and early medical advice is specially important in the case of babies and small children. They could collapse very quickly.

Many elderly people have a relatively low sense of thirst and they too need special attention. Encourage and coax them to drink adequately to replace fluid lost through diarrhoea and vomiting.

Do not allow remnants of the suspected food to be thrown away. Put them safely aside for the doctor may wish to see them and to send them for laboratory tests.

Fevers with Sweating

Very high fevers and sweating, as for instance a malarial attack, are accompanied by a very weakening loss of fluids and minerals (see p. 175). The same principles of giving salty drinks apply as for diarrhoea and vomiting.

Toothache

The only effective treatment for toothache is to see a dentist. In the meantime a helpful first-aid measure is to apply a small pledget of wool soaked in oil of cloves. But do not use this more than three times in the day and try to keep the oil from running on the gum.

Let the patient take any pain-relieving tablets to which he is accustomed.

Hiccups

Hiccups are usually harmless and it is only rarely that they persist so long that a doctor's help is needed. But while they last they can be a great nuisance, annoying and embarrassing the sufferer. As he inhales his diaphragm goes into sharp muscular spasm and the opening of the voice box (larynx) at the upper end of his airway closes abruptly. A sudden block to air inflow produces the jerky cough-like sound.

A number of things can start the attack: very hot or spicy foods and drinks, alcohol, eating too much and too fast, or exercising after a large meal are some of them. Once hiccups have started, a psychological factor sometimes keeps them going.

Tradition has advised all sorts of treatments such as swallowing dry bread or crushed ice, pulling on the tongue or even pressing on the eyeballs. If they succeed it probably is because they allow the victim to relax in the belief that something is being done to help him.

There are two methods with a more scientific approach. Hard pressure against the diaphragm may stop its repeated spasms. This can be done by the sufferer lying down on his back, bending his knees against his abdomen and pressing them there for a few seconds by gripping the back of his thighs.

Less acrobatic and more convenient is using the dampening-down effect of carbon dioxide on the activity of nerves, which stimulate hiccuping. Let the patient spend a little time rebreathing the air he exhales, which contains a relatively high level of carbon dioxide. Tell him to breathe in and out of a large paper bag with its opening held firmly round his nose and mouth. Please note that he should **not** use a plastic bag, which could fold up against and cling to his mouth and nostrils.

Adhering Skin

There are two, quite different, circumstances that could make skin stick so hard to an object that it risks being torn if separation is attempted by pulling away.

Extreme cold

This may (for instance) freeze the fingers and palm of a hand on to a grasped metal object. Or a child may put its lip against an object in a freezer cabinet and find it stuck.

Let the patient stay still and avoid pulling while you quickly seek warm (not hot) water to pour between the object and the skin.

Modern adhesives

Some of these bond in seconds and can cause difficulties if accidentally they get on to skin. On no account should any stuck skin surface be pulled away. Get the area immersed in warm soapy water and then use a thin blunt edge (like a teaspoon's handle) to roll or peel the surfaces apart.

If an eye is involved wash it with warm water and apply a covering pad. Then the patient must wait without trying to force the lids open or to manipulate the eye. There will be a heavy flow of tear fluid, which will clear the adhesive away within one to four days.

Questions

1. A weeping, distraught woman runs from a bus, which has stopped outside a busy chemist's shop. She opens the door and goes behind the counter to the dispenser crying that on the bus she has suddenly become completely blind. What should the dispenser do?

2. Briefly describe the essential differences between the causes of acute heart failure, of coronary thrombosis and of angina.

3. In a crowded fairground a pale and dazed-looking man is lurching along clumsily. He bumps into you, touches you with a sweaty, trembling hand and speaks, but you cannot understand what he says. What might be the matter and how could you deal with it?

4. A small crowd is looking down on a man who is lying on the ground alongside a wall. As you approach he begins sharp jerking of arms and legs. What can you expect to happen next and how can you protect him?

5. Your grandmother excuses herself for being late at breakfast explaining that a headache bothers her. She walks badly with one foot shuffling and she is clumsy, spilling tea on her chin and neck as she tries to drink. What should be done?

6. Returning from a train's buffet a commuter finds a stranger in his compartment. He is crouched in a corner seat, pale and struggling to get his breath, making harsh, wheezy noises. The only other passenger puffs unconcernedly at his pipe saying he does not know what to do. The commuter is wiser; describe his actions.

7. While you are visiting your bachelor uncle he begins to look uneasy. Falling back, pale and weak, he clutches at his chest, which, he says, is painful. He tries to get up to look for aspirin. How can you help him?

19
Emergency Childbirth

The average length of a pregnancy is 40 weeks after the date of the last period. If a pregnant woman begins vaginal bleeding before the likely time of the baby's birth, she may be having a miscarriage or a premature labour. These terms need defining. A *miscarriage* describes a delivery when the baby is too small to be likely to survive. This is considered to be up to the twenty-fourth week of pregnancy. The word *abortion* means the same thing but in general it is used when the event has been deliberately created. However *spontaneous abortion* is the medical term for the misfortune of a miscarriage, which happens without planning, without interference.

Miscarriage

Vaginal bleeding may be quite slight. Put the patient to rest, in bed, if possible. Let her be relaxed with her head on pillows and her knees a little bent. Put a sanitary towel (or a small clean towel) over the vulva. Call a doctor at once or send her by ambulance to hospital. The situation is generally more urgent if she has pains.

Heavy bleeding is very urgent too. In this case she could develop shock, and you should have her lying with her head low (p. 105).

If she passes any clots or solid matter, keep these for the doctor to examine. If she needs to pass urine she should use a chamber rather than a lavatory pan, so as to avoid losing anything she passes.

Childbirth

Generally the mother's first symptoms of the onset of labour are a low backache and abdominal cramp like a pain or discomfort. There is also a discharge from the vagina of a little, bloodstained mucus. Ask the mother about her doctor and the arrangements planned for the delivery. At this point there should be time to follow these plans.

The length of labour

The times given below for the different stages of labour are average ones under normal circumstances. As you will see they allow a good chance for expert help to become available. However you must bear in mind that the cases with which the first aider has to deal are very often labours that proceed far quicker than the average. There is one very real comfort you can give to the mother and to yourself: such rapid labours are likely to be straightforward.

Who delivers the baby?

The truth is that you do not deliver the baby; the mother delivers the baby. You are a gentle, non-interfering, guide. Important as they are, your actions are only to assist a natural process.

Only in some unlikely circumstances would you have to do more. These are the passages in italics in the following account. It would be helpful for you to study these pages twice. First read only the parts in ordinary type; then re-read them, this time taking in the italicised passages as well.

First Preparations

1. The mother, especially if it is her first baby, may be very anxious. Help her by acting calmly and confidently, reassuring her that labour generally and successfully looks after itself. Although you arrange for her privacy, she may wish to have a woman friend or relative by her side and also, perhaps, her husband.

2. A full bladder can impede delivery. Let the mother pass urine, using a chamber and not the lavatory pan.

3. Warm the room.

4. The bed will have one pillow, a couple of blankets and a clean sheet. If possible put something like plastic or mackintosh sheeting under the bed sheet. You can use towels or clean paper as a substitute for the sheets.

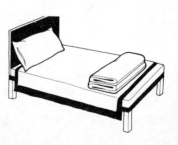

5. Wash your hands and forearms very thoroughly, with good nail scrubbing. At various stages of the delivery repeat this so that your hands remain scrupulously clean.

6. Sterilise a pair of scissors and four pieces of string or strong tape 25

cm (10 in.) long by boiling them for
ten minutes in a saucepan of water.
Leave them to cool in the saucepan
with its lid on.

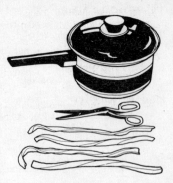

7. Get together a clean basin,
holding clean swabs of gauze or
cotton wool (or, failing these, a
number of clean handkerchiefs). Also
have handy a receptacle into which
you can throw used swabs. Prepare
pads of clean cloth, which, at the time
of the baby's birth, will cover the back
passage of the mother.

8. Have two clean thick towels
ready, one for the mother and one for
the baby.

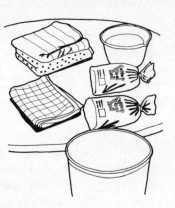

All this implies the usual domestic
comforts. Precipitately fast labour
could happen in totally inappropriate
places (e.g. during a country walk or
in a car). The first aider copes by
improvising as best as he can and by
trying to send an urgent message for a
doctor or an ambulance.

The Labour Contractions; the First Stage

As labour progresses the mother is likely to feel intermittent
contractions ('pains') in the abdomen. They are due to activity of the
uterus (womb) which is preparing itself and its opening for moving out
the baby. In the average labour this first stage lasts 12 to 16 hours (or
less if the mother has had a baby previously). Contractions are spaced
out at 10 to 15 minutes intervals; each may last 30 to 90 seconds.

Encourage the mother to be as relaxed as possible during the
contractions, for tension can hinder progress. She need not be in bed;
she may walk about as long as she is not too uncomfortable.

The Labour Contractions: the Second Stage

Once the opening of the uterus has widened enough to let the baby
through, contractions become more forceful and frequent coming
every 1 to 5 minutes. The muscular wall of the uterus is beginning to
push the baby down and out. In the average labour this stage lasts one
hour or less.

Prepare the mother for the birth by having her lie on her back with her head and shoulders comfortably on the pillow. Her lower clothes are off, but she is kept warm by blankets over the abdomen and chest. She should keep her knees bent and falling outwards with her feet well apart on the bed. Place a towel under her buttocks. Keep a cloth over the back passage to protect the vulva from becoming soiled.

Now the mother feels she cannot relax but wants to tense her abdominal muscles and to 'bear down' and push with each contraction. Let her do this. It will be more effective if, at the beginning of the contraction, she takes a deep breath in and holds it and if she grasps her knees as she pushes. But advise her to relax completely and to breathe deeply between the contractions.

At some point in the labour the membranes holding the fluid in which the baby lies will rupture. There is a sudden flow or gush of watery liquid from the vagina. This could startle the mother, but reassure her that it is quite normal.

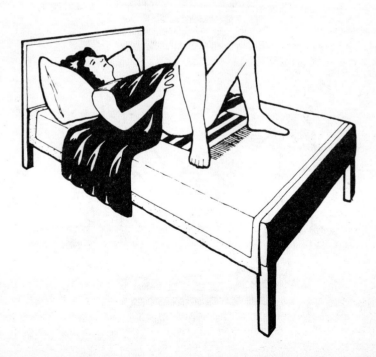

The Birth of the Head

The second stage of contractions continues until the baby is born. Each contraction pushes the baby down a little further, and the top of its head, dark and wet, will appear at the vulva (A). Gradually the vulva will be distended (although the head may recede a little between each contraction).

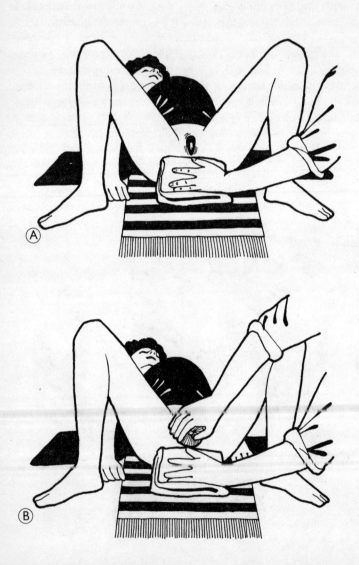

As the full width of the head seems about to come through, you should try to avoid its doing so with a sudden spurt that could harm the baby and the mother. During the next contraction cup your hand lightly over the head. Do not aim to hold it back, but only to steady its emergence (B). At the same time ask the mother to take deep panting breaths during the contraction; this will reduce the strength of her 'bearing down', making your control of the head easier.

You may find that it takes more than this one contraction to get the head fully out. When this has happened support it lightly with one hand underneath it.

Very rarely the membranes holding the liquid in which the baby lies do not rupture spontaneously during labour. If a membrane covers the baby's head tear it with your fingers, push it away from the nose and mouth and let the liquid escape. Otherwise the baby could asphyxiate when it tries to draw its first breath.

The Birth of the Baby's Body

Support the head with one hand underneath. With a finger of the other hand check whether the umbilical cord lies around the neck (C). The cord feels knobbly and rubbery. It holds the blood vessels by which the baby (at this stage of its life) gets its oxygen supply. *If you do find the*

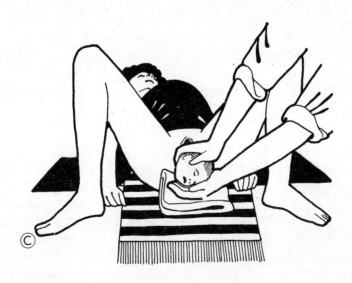

cord around the neck use the hooked finger to ease it gently over the head, so that it does not tighten when the rest of the baby is born with the next contractions.

Still supporting the head wait for the next contractions. They will get the shoulders through and then the rest of the baby will follow. As it comes, guide and lift it by holding it under the armpits—but do **not** pull. And be very careful for the baby is slippery to handle.

Once the baby is fully out keep it sloping with the head downwards, so that fluid and mucus can run out of the mouth and nose. Gently mop these parts with gauze.

The baby looks dusky or blue until it gives a cry and begins to breathe, when it becomes pinker.

If after two minutes it does not breathe give Artificial Respiration in very gentle puffs (p. 136) keeping the head low.

Once it starts breathing, wrap a towel round it and let it lie on the mother or by her side.

In all your handling of the baby be careful not to pull on, or stretch the umbilical cord, which is still partly inside the mother. Its other end is attached to the placenta (the 'afterbirth').

Delivering the Placenta ('After-birth')

The placenta is still inside the uterus. Within the next fifteen minutes further contractions of the uterus will detach it and push it out; some slight bleeding accompanies this. Ask the mother to help by 'bearing down' well with the contractions. (They are less strong than the ones that got the baby out).

She can help also, by putting the newborn child to the breast. Sucking action on the nipple reflexly strengthens the contractions of the uterus.

Once the placenta is out put a sanitary towel or clean pad over the vulva.

If bleeding is heavy this could be due to inadequate contractions of the uterus. Encourage them to get stronger by gently rubbing (not pushing) the top of the uterus through the abdominal wall: you can feel it at about the level of the navel. Maintain this rubbing until bleeding decreases.

Should bleeding become very severe, treat the mother as for shock (p. 105) with her head low and, if possible, raising the foot of the bed.

The Umbilical Cord

Now you have the baby and the placenta delivered, with the umbilical cord linking the two. If medical help is likely to come soon, leave the cord alone.

However if no help will be available you have to cut the cord and separate the baby from the placenta. Wait for ten minutes after the birth (during which time some of the placenta's blood enters the baby). Before cutting you must tie the cord to prevent bleeding. Use three of the strings or tapes you have sterilised. Tie the first one 15 cm (6 in.) from the baby, and the second and third each 5 cm (2 in.) from the preceding ones. Make really secure reef knots (p. 16) but take care not to pull on the cord as you do this.

With the sterilised scissors, cut between the second and third knots. There will be two knots on the cord attached to the baby and one on that attached to the placenta. Put a clean dressing over the cut end of the baby's cord.

Keep the placenta in a plastic bag for the doctor or midwife to examine later.

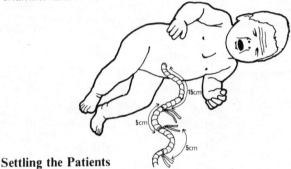

Settling the Patients

Do **not** wash the baby. Place it, wrapped in its towel, on its side in a cot. It should lie flat, and **not** have a pillow. In the absence of a cot use a deep basket, clean box or drawer lined by towels. Do not allow the baby to get cold.

About ten minutes after you tied the cord look under the dressing over the cut end to make sure there is no bleeding. If there is you must tie another knot using the fourth string or tape.

Make sure the mother is comfortable and let her have something to drink like tea or cocoa.

Postscript

The whole of labour is a special example of the importance of repeated, confident, reassuring talk to the patient. Let the mother know what is happening and not feel 'lost' at the far end of the action.

Questions

1. Describe the bed arrangements for an emergency delivery. During the birth of the baby what should be the position of the mother?

2. In the delivery of the baby two different stages of contractions are described. What are they and their effects? During the second stage how do you advise the mother to help herself?

3. How do you protect the baby's head as it is being born? And how do you protect the baby's breathing after it has been born?

4. A few minutes after the baby has been delivered and before the delivery of the placenta there is heavy bleeding from the vagina. What do you do?

5. The baby and the placenta have been delivered. Under what circumstances should you separate them? And how do you do this?

6. About three months after her last period a woman has colicky pains and seeks some medicine for her 'indigestion'. What might you suspect and what questions should you ask?

20
Traffic Accidents

Car and motorcycle accidents give special problems in addition to the injuries they cause. You not only have to help the patient but also may have to cope with a potentially dangerous road situation.

Approaching the Scene

If you are in a car yourself do not drive right up to the damaged vehicle. Park a little way off, leaving room for ambulance and rescue services to move in close when they arrive. If you can do so safely (to yourself and to others) park off the road on the verge. At least park as close to the road edge as you can. Switch on your hazard lights if you have them.

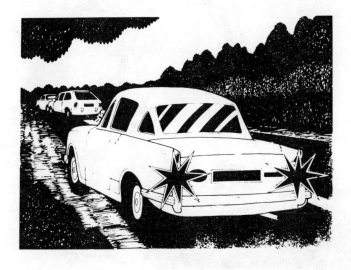

At night time have your headlights directed to the scene, without blinding drivers of other cars on the road. Put on your brakes and switch off your engine. Switch on your hazard lights, if you have them.

Coping with the First Emergencies

Quickly assess the injured. Look for the priorities:

1. Those who have ceased breathing and need artificial respiration (p. 131).
2 Those who have an obstructed airway (p. 41).
3. Those whose severe bleeding needs immediate control (p. 27).

Give immediate aid but try not to move the victims if you can possibly avoid it. Mouth-to-mouth artificial respiration to someone in a car is inconvenient and could be difficult but in most cases you can do it.

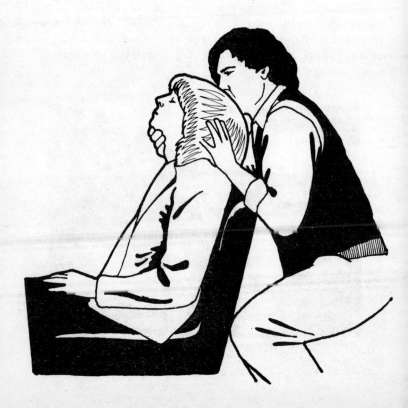

Also you can carefully correct and then maintain the position of the head of an unconscious person, extending it back, but not letting it twist or turn if there is a risk of fractured spine in the neck. Alternatively the improvised collar described on p. 89 makes an excellent safeguard. Clear any vomit or blood from the mouth. By these actions you not only protect the spine at the neck but also safeguard the patient's airway.

Pressure on a severely bleeding wound is generally easy. Do not hesitate to cut clothing to reach the wound. Rapidly improvise the necessary pad and bandage from any material to hand.

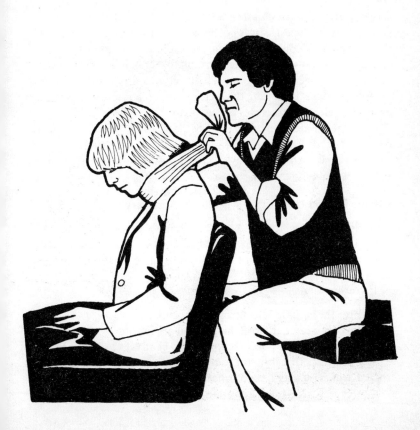

Look for Other Victims

In collisions it is not unusual for a victim to be thrown some distance. Ask a conscious passenger how many there were in the car. With motorcycles think of the possibility that there was a pillion rider. Quickly explore behind a low wall or hedge or in a ditch for the hidden casualty. If possible send bystanders to do this for you. Remember also that some dazed people may wander away from the accident scene.

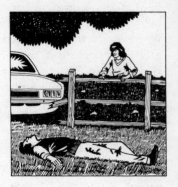

Leave Victims in the Car

It is rarely necessary to get the patient out of the car before the rescue services arrive. If bystanders want to do this, tell them to desist. Getting out of modern cars is not always easy for the agile and healthy; the movements could grossly increase damage to the injured. In collisions car walls often crumple up and fold closely around the driver and his passengers. When the rescue services arrive they will have protective means of getting the victims out, even if this means cutting away the vehicle's structures about them.

Unless there are many men (and perhaps also machinery) properly organised to do this, it is unwise to try to lift a car that is pinning someone down. An attempt by too few people may fail, so that the car falls back doing greater harm.

Get the Injured Out only if Absolutely Necessary

Fire risk, noxious fumes in the car and the need to give chest compression when the heart is not beating are cases where you have urgently to break the rule of leaving the injured in the car.

If you are alone:

1. Free the casualty's feet from the pedals.
2. Fold his nearer arm over his abdomen; slip your forearm under his nearer armpit and support his chin so as to bend his head straight back.
3. Slip your other forearm round his back and grasp the wrist of his folded arm. You may have to rotate him on his seat to manage this.
4. Keep his head fully supported against your shoulder and slide the

patient out of the door. Drag him a safe distance.

5. Lie him on the ground by flattening yourself down, taking care to manoeuvre your knee away from his body.

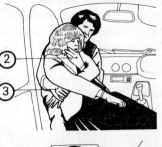

6. Very gently free his folded arm. Throughout you will be extremely careful to keep his head bent backwards and to avoid its turning.

If you have someone to help, you let him stand on the other side of the patient. He gets his arms and hands under the buttocks and legs, supporting them, as you draw the patient out of the car.

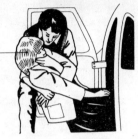

Now place the patient in the Recovery Position, unless his injuries preclude this. In that case someone will have to maintain the head position to guard the airway.

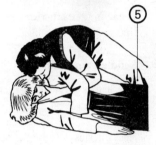

Safeguards against Further Dangers

1. Do not allow anyone on the scene to smoke. Petrol may have been spilled.

2. If the vehicle runs on diesel fuel you may find an outside switch that cuts off the fuel.

3. Switch off the ignition of the damaged car, if it is still on. If you can, disconnect the battery. Fires could start if the electric circuit is active.

4. Apply the brake. If the brake lever is not functioning and the car is on a slope, put something large (stone, box, removable seat from your own car) behind a wheel to prevent the car moving down.

5. If smoke is rising from the engine use a fire extinguisher. (Your car ought to carry, as a matter of course, an extinguisher of the specialised type for use on engines. A practical point is that the cost of replacement to your used extinguisher will generally be borne by the company insuring the accident car.) In the absence of an extinguisher, smother the smouldering part with earth or with a rug.

6. Another item, which you should have in your car, is the reflecting

red triangle to be set on the road about 200 m (220 yd) behind or beyond the accident scene as a warning to approaching drivers. This is particularly important at night, or round a bend in the road. Use bystanders to do this, and use them also to wave down approaching cars.

7. At night time those helping should carry or wear something white (large handkerchief, newspaper) so that their presence can be seen.

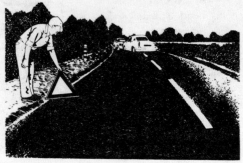

A car in contact with electric wires
See p. 127.

Sending for Help

Use a messenger if you can, or call upon the drivers of other cars to find the nearest telephone, perhaps in a nearby house. In Britain dialling 999 gets the telephone exchange's immediate response, and the caller asks to be connected to the ambulance service. The message must give very clearly the exact site of the accident (and any helpful landmarks), the number of injured, the estimated nature of the injuries, whether anyone is trapped and also what sort of vehicles are involved. If a tanker containing dangerous chemicals is involved report the information given on its hazard warning (see p. 218).

It is not necessary to telephone the police as well, for the ambulance office will do this for you.

Additional First Aid

You have now, as rapidly as you could, dealt with the most urgent features of the accident. While awaiting the arrival of ambulance and police deal with the secondary points of first aid. You will, by now, have been able to get out the first-aid kit, which should be an integral part of your own car's equipment. Dress any open wounds; immobilise as best you can any obvious fractures, which you can reach without moving the patient; cover the patient with a rug, coat or a metal foil blanket (see p. 185) to prevent his losing heat. Keep up the patient's morale by being both methodical and reassuring. Let him know that an ambulance is coming.

If any bystander is excitedly shouting or acting in some way to dismay your patient even further, try to detail a suitable person to calm him down and to draw him away.

Do not 'tidy up' the accident scene by moving debris and other objects, unless they constitute a danger where they lie. The position of these items may prove to be important evidence when the police try to assess the cause of the accident.

The Motor Cyclist's Helmet

Loosen the chin strap for it could be pressing awkwardly. The helmet itself is best left on unless special circumstances like fatal injuries needing immediate attention dictate that it should come off. Also it ought to be removed speedily if it is interfering with breathing or if the casualty is vomiting.

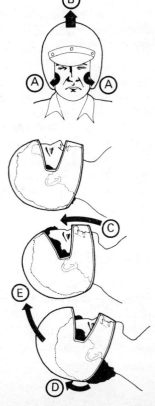

If it is possible and easy for him let the casualty himself take it off. If you have to do the removing:

1. Undo the strap under the chin.
2. Get a helper to steady the casualty's head and neck firmly, with his hands just beneath the lower end of the helmet.
3. With your two hands ease outwards the lower edges of the helmet so that they are not pressing against the sides of the head (A).
4. If the helmet is one that covers only the upper part of the head slip it off by moving it up and back (B).

If the helmet is a full-face one you must get the chin cover off first. Tilt the helmet backwards until the chin is clear (C). Then do the opposite motion, tilting the helmet forwards, free of the lower part of the back of the head (D) and slide it up and off (E).

All the while your helper is supporting the casualty's head and preventing it from moving.

Your Car's First-aid Kit

See p. 228.

The Motorway Accident

Because of the traffic's speed it is dangerous to stop on the carriageway; there is too great a risk of being caught in further crashes from fast cars coming up.

Stop on the hard shoulder a wise distance behind the accident scene. Put on your hazard lights, if you have them. Run along the hard shoulder to the nearest telephone to alert the police. Telephones are about a mile apart and signs on the marker posts show the direction of the nearest one.

Dangerous Loads

Some tankers contain chemicals, which, on escaping, could mean danger to those who approach. They carry large 'hazard warning' panels which, by international regulations, give coded information—standardised in many countries.

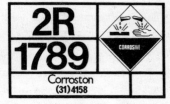

On the right-hand side there is a diamond with wording and symbol to show the type of material, such as radioactive, corrosive, explosive, inflammable, and so on. On the left are code letters and numbers indicating what the material is and the methods needed to cope with it. The lower area gives the name of the manufacturer and a telephone number from which specialist advice can be obtained.

These codes are for use by the emergency rescue services, but the 'hazard warning' itself is prominently visible to everyone.

When there is any involvement with dangerous material your role is to notify the police fast. Stay well clear and make sure others do so too. This may seem a harsh decision if you want to attend to victims in, or near, the tanker, but is justified by the risks of fire, explosion or poisonous fumes.

Questions

1. Rarely there are occasions when you should stand back and limit yourself to calling the rescue services instead of going to help in a road accident. What are they?

2. As you, and your friend, come round the bend of a country lane you find a motorcycle lying on the road. Some distance from it the motor cyclist, still helmeted, is lying on the ground. He is unconscious and blood is coming from his mouth. What do you do?

3. A closed saloon car has skidded on a hill and hit a tree, crumpling its bonnet. The driver is conscious; he has a large, freely bleeding, gash on the forehead and he complains of pain in the right knee. Before sending for help what actions do you take, and in what order?

4. How would you send for help to a car smash? What details should you include in the message?

5. What are the circumstances which would justify removing an occupant from a smashed car before the rescue services arrive? How would you get him out?

21
Giving Drinks

Throughout the study of first aid the point is made that you should give nothing by mouth to the severly injured patient. He may become unconscious; he may vomit. Also he may vomit while unconscious or semi-conscious and some of the material brought up could move chokingly into the windpipe.

The patient could need an operation and anaesthetic, again with the possibility of vomiting. Anaesthetists do have measures of protecting the windpipe but, in general, it is far preferable for the patient's stomach to be empty during an operation.

There are exceptions to the 'no drink' teaching. Burns, crush injuries, poisoning, heat exhaustion, hypothermia and low sugar levels in the treated diabetic are examples. A few quite simple rules apply:

1. Never try to give a drink to the unconscious or barely conscious person. He must be co-operatively able to swallow to avoid the risk of choking.

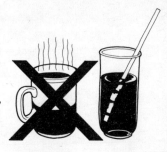

2. Never, under any circumstances, give alcohol. The idea that brandy (for instance) revives and supports is quite false.

3. If the drink is to be a hot one, do not give it too hot. The enfeebled patient offered really steaming fluid is likely to reject it after the first scorching sip. Let the drink be comfortably warm.

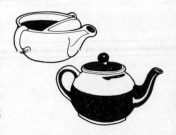

4. If the patient is lying down do not present him with a cup or mug filled to the top. The fluid will flow down his chin on to his chest. Make sure the container is only two-thirds full.

5. A drink may be taken through a straw. Or you may use the usefully-shaped invalid feeding cup with its spout and its top front guard. If none is available a small teapot makes an excellent substitute.

6. Do not let the patient drink in large gulps. He should take small, repeated, and frequent sips.

22
Coping with Emergencies

Instruction in first-aid books and classes is (hopefully) simple and easy to understand, although the real emergency can prove messy and confusing. Teaching the principles is generally based on the concept of a single casualty in a straightforward situation. However, the chapter on traffic accidents considered having to cope with several victims at a scene of potential danger. Such problems can occur in many other first-aid events.

A planned system allows you to act fast and methodically under most circumstances.

Avoid Danger

How safe are the surroundings? Could you become the next casualty? Beware of fire, smoke (p. 92), fumes, electricity (pp. 126–7), structures likely to collapse, dangerous chemicals (p. 218) and fast, uncontrollable traffic. Do not rush in carelessly. Quickly, calmly, assess the scene before you enter it.

The Priority Patient

When several patients are injured do not automatically attend to the nearest. Make a speedy survey and judgement as to who, most urgently, needs help. Priority goes to.

keeping the patients' airways clear (p. 49);
resuscitation where breathing and heart beat have stopped (p. 130);
controlling heavy bleeding (p. 27);
Recovery Position for the unconscious person who can be moved (p. 112).

A shouting or crying victim is likely to be in far less danger than one who is silent and unconscious.

Treat the Injured where you Find Them

Do not move the patient until you know it is safe to do so. This is specially important if the injuries could include a fracture. One of your early tasks may have to be preventing a hurt and fallen patient from struggling up or well-meaning bystanders from trying to help him to his feet.

Exceptionally a particularly risky setting may force you to break this rule so that both you and patient get out of danger quickly.

Keep the Area Safe

Ensure a safe working scene as soon as it is practicable to do this. An accident can produce a number of hazards lying around. Get such things as fallen ladders, broken glass, moveable obstructions or spilt liquids out of the way.

But if the accident is one likely to be followed by police enquiries, move objects as little as possible and note their original positions. Their disposition, and even the pattern of blood stains, could be important evidence.

Be Informed

Unless an obvious emergency makes you take immediate action, spend very brief time getting details of what happened. Jumping to conclusions may make you miss an important injury. *Get the history*: ask the patient or bystanders what happened. *Learn the symptoms*: ask the patient what he feels, where he has pain or handicap. *Obtain the signs*: make a careful, methodical examination to see, feel, and hear abnormal features. These could include such things as pallor, deformed limbs, wet patches of clothes over bleeding sites, swellings, bruises, unequal pupils, harsh breathing or any of the possible clues about the patient's condition.

Cards, necklet or bracelet inscriptions are carried by some patients to give information about conditions that might make them need emergency treatment. Examples are diabetes, epilepsy, allergies and special drugs prescribed.

Physical First Aid

Clearing the airway, resuscitating, stopping heavy bleeding and the use of the Recovery Position have already been marked as the priorities. Then attention goes to the following—more or less in this order:

dressing wounds (p. 2);
immobilising fractures (p. 70);
positioning the patient correctly (pp. 52, 105);
protecting him against shock (p. 105), including covering him.

Undress the patient as little as possible. If you do have to remove a coat or shirt, begin by clearing it back from neck and shoulders and getting the sleeve off an uninjured arm; then slide off the other sleeve, trying not to move the arm it covers. If you have to get the patient's trousers off first undo the waist band and front and bring them down to thigh level.

Sometimes to avoid moving the patient dangerously, you will have to cut clothing. As far as possible let this be along seam lines.

Do not leave a patient unguarded unless this is absolutely unavoidable. The unconscious patient may vomit or his breathing may fail. He may partly come to and need gentle restraining from moving. The conscious patient after severe injury can, understandably, feel miserably anxious if left alone.

Mental First Aid

The importance of your psychological approach has been mentioned in the chapter on shock. Emotion is a very potent intensifier of physical reactions. Fear will not cause shock but could considerably aggravate it. In the same way medical emergencies like severe heart or asthmatic attacks can be worsened by the patient's anxiety. Occasionally calm reassurance can be life-saving.

You need to reassure carefully. Never depart from truth in the attempt to calm a patient. For instance, if you know for certain that he has a fracture do not conceal this from him, should he ask. He (and his companions) will lose faith in you and your statements when the facts come out.

Present truths in a way that will help his morale. For instance, you reply that, yes, you believe he has a broken bone, and at the same time you explain that you have now stopped bleeding, covered the wound and protected the fracture so as to put it in the best state for full treatment by the specialists. Your remarks will always stress the positive and helpful facts about himself or his companion or, indeed, about his motorcycle which lies bent on the ground alongside him.

Never whisper to anyone near the patient (who will fear the worst). Let all your statements in front of him be clear and encouraging. Should you have to say something that might cause anxiety move out of his hearing first.

Do not think that someone apparently unconscious will not hear what goes on around him. He may well be able to register (and to regret) anything he overhears.

If you have to deal at the same time with one anxiously speaking and shouting (but relatively unharmed), patient and one unconscious patient, reassure the first one that you will be with him very soon, as you go to look after the second.

Your calmness, method, and attitude of confidence can contribute greatly to the help you offer. Some victims of accidents become dazed and uncertain. Such people welcome and respond well to clearly given instructions.

On the other hand, patients could be depressed by the morbid staring and careless comments of bystanders.

Bystanders

Get rid of bystanders pressing around the casualty for a better view. Do this by ordering rather than by pleading. You have already established that as a first aider you are in charge; people will be prepared to obey if you tell them firmly to stand back from the patient and 'give him air'. (That air is already reaching him is immaterial.)

Some may help in tidying up the area under your directions. You can get a volubly anxious bystander off the scene by asking him to do a task, like looking for some marginally useful equipment.

But use the quiet, dependable-looking bystander who is willing to help. Give him clear instructions if he is to handle the patient. Or choose him to be your messenger in sending for help.

Sending for Help

Generally, for serious cases, calling out a doctor is less useful than sending for an ambulance. A doctor may be out visiting patients at home or hospital; his equipment for dealing with major injuries is likely to be less specific and more limited than that of an ambulance; very often, even the finest doctor cannot do more at the accident scene than can the good first aider.

If you send for help by telephone choose a trustworthy messenger. Write down the message and be sure he understands it. In Britain he will dial 999 and ask the operator for the ambulance service. When he is put through he will detail:

the nature of the accident and of the injuries;
the number and sex of the casualties and (if this is relevant) their ages;
the exact address or location; with guiding details.

At night time it might be difficult for an ambulance driver or doctor to find your home. You could have a look-out in the street to stand and guide. Or you could make the house very obvious by pulling back all front-room curtains, opening the front door and switching all the lights on.

You may wish to drive a patient to hospital yourself. Think twice before you do this with a severely injured person. Might he collapse on the way? Would your car space let you put him in the Recovery Position? Would you have someone else in the car to help? How much does it matter that your car could not have the speed and traffic priority allowed to ambulances?

Afterwards

After you have completed first aid, and as you wait for help, continue to speak quietly but encouragingly to the patient. Get his name and address and tell him who you are.

If necessary get also the name of a relative or friend whom he wishes to be told of his state. In most cases, however, it is wise to leave this task of informing in the very capable hands of the police or hospital authorities.

Write a brief account of what you found and what you did; give it to the ambulance attendant to pass on to the hospital. Also hand over to him any personal property of the patient.

Rarely the first aider is called on to give evidence about the event, possibly in a legal enquiry. This can happen several weeks or months afterwards when memory may well be poor.

If you think there is any likelihood that, long after your first-aid help, you will be subjected to incisive cross-examination, write a detailed record of the time, place, people and injuries, exactly what you did, and of your opinion of the patient's condition. It could prove invaluable were you questioned. On the other hand you might never need it—except to remind you, gratifyingly, of the good, perhaps life-saving, service you once provided.

23
First-Aid Kits

The essence of first aid is to be able to improvise from what you can find on the scene in an emergency. However for the home and for the car it is right to have ready a planned kit to which you can immediately turn.

A jumble of ill-wrapped bits of dressing loosely held in polythene or paper bags does not deserve the name of a first-aid kit. Keep the material in a clearly labelled box, which you use for nothing else. The ideal box should be firm and easily cleaned and have a closely-fitting lid; make sure it is of tin or of plastic, as is used in freezer cabinets.

When you have decided on the contents stick a list detailing them inside the lid. Each dressing should be in its own closed packet. Once a packet has been opened discard any unused material and replace the packet at the first opportunity.

For the Home

Keep the box in a place known to all members of the household, but inaccessible to children. Avoid its being subjected to a steamy atmosphere as in the bathroom or by the kitchen sink.

Suggested contents:

Small paper tissues: one pack;
Cotton wool 15g pack: one;
White gauze 1 m pack: one;
Adhesive strapping 2½ cm wide: one roll;
Adhesive dressing strip 5 cm wide (see p. 14): one;
P.F.A. dressings 5 cm square and 10 cm square (see p. 11): one of each;
Plain bandages 5 cm and 7½ cm wide: one of each;
Conforming or elastic bandage 7½ cm wide (see p. 12): one;
Tubular gauze bandage, small size, with applicator (see p. 14): one;
Prepared sterile dressings, medium and large sizes (see p. 14): one of

each;

> Oil of cloves (see p. 199): one very small bottle;
> Safety pins: 4;
> Scissors (blunt ended): one pair;
> Tweezers: one pair.

This kit is not to be confused with a home medicine cabinet. It is designed to give first aid to injuries only. The one exception is oil of cloves, which can temporarily ease toothache, while awaiting the dentist's treatment.

For the Car

Your car should hold three important accessory items (see p. 215):

> A large standing torch. Check its batteries at frequent intervals;
> A warning red triangle;
> A fire extinguisher, suitable for use on car engines.

Wounds in road accidents can be fairly big and the contents of your box reflects this:

> Cotton wool 15 g packs: two;
> White gauze 1 metre pack: two;
> Adhesive strapping $2\frac{1}{2}$ cm wide: one roll;
> Adhesive dressing strip $7\frac{1}{2}$ cm wide: one;
> P.F.A. dressings (see p. 11): 10 cm square and 10×20 cm: one of each;
> Plain bandages: 5 cm and $7\frac{1}{2}$ cm wide: two of each;
> Conforming or elastic bandage $7\frac{1}{2}$ cm wide (see p. 12): two;
> Prepared sterile dressings, large size (see p. 14): two;
> Safety pins: six;
> Scissors—a large size capable of cutting clothing: one pair;
> Rescue blanket (see p. 185): one;
> Notebook and pencil for messages.

It would be realistic to add to this a ready-made 'improvised' neck splint created out of a folded newspaper within a woman's stocking as described on p. 89.

Answers to Questions

Try first to answer as fully as possible (preferably in writing) before using the book to check up.

Chapter 1. Wounds

1. Crush injury (major type). Follow treatment on pp. 8 and 9.
2. Dress wound as for embedded object (pp. 2–4). Advise patient about tetanus protection (p.9).
3. Pattern bruise with possibility of internal injury. Check for possible fracture and patient's general condition. Advise a medical check. (p. 7).
4. Antiseptics are only for the rare application of 'second aid'. Should be used carefully (p. 4).

Chapter 2. Dressings and Bandages

1. Cover plus pad plus bandage; improvization (pp. 12, 14); adhesive dressing (p. 14); tubular gauze bandage (p. 14).
2. See pp.13 and 23.
3. Improvization of dressings (pp. 12 and 14) and of sling (p. 20).
4. See pp. 12, 13 and 23.

Chapter 3. Blood and Bleeding

1. Suspect stomach bleeding. See p. 35.
2. See pp. 31 and 32.
3. See pp. 24 and 26.
4. Follow principles described on pp. 28 and 29.
5. See p. 33.

Chapter 4. Lungs and Breathing

1. The patient needs a medical check. See p. 47.
2. See p. 49.
3. See pp. 39–41.

4. See pp. 50 and 52.

5. Follow him; advise him; See p. 41. If necessary act as on pp. 42–7.

Chapter 5. Joints and Muscles

1. See p. 51.

2. See p. 60.

3. Sprains relate to joints and their ligaments; strains relate to muscles. Compare the treatments on pp. 60 and 61.

4. Suspect a hernia (see p. 62).

5. See illustration pp. 57 and 67.

Chapter 6. Fractures; General Principles

1. See p. 68.

2. See pp. 65 and 66.

3. Prevent dangerous moving (see p. 70). Look for and control severe bleeding (see pp. 27 and 70).

4. See p. 65. An indirect fracture may be missed if not considered.

Chapter 7. Fractures; specific sites

1. See pages 76–8.

2. Suspect fracture spine at the neck. Follow principles on p. 87–9.

3. Risks of choking; see p. 74.

4. Possible fracture of thigh bone or of pelvis. See pp. 79–82.

5. The patient may show the characteristic head tilt and be supporting the arm on the injured side (see p. 76).

Chapter 8. Burns

1. See pp. 94–6.

2. See pp. 92

3. See p. 98.

4. The wider the burn area the greater are the likely loss of plasma and the consequent risk of shock (see p. 92).

Chapter 9. Shock

1. p. 105–8

2. P. 108.

3. Pp. 106 and 107.

4. Pp. 102–4.

5. Pp. 100–2. In injuries the common factor causing shock is loss of blood from the circulation.

Chapter 10. The Unconscious Person
1. See p. 115.
2. Preventing careless moving of the patient because of possible fractured spine (see p. 111).
3. See p. 112; (*a*) ensures stability; (*b*) ensures a clear airway.
4. Guard his airway by removing pillows and extending his head back (see p. 110).
5. Where the movement would aggravate a suspected fracture, especially in the spine (see p. 87 and 112).

Chapter 11. Head and Brain
1. See p. 122.
2. Disquieting; suggests increasing compression. See p. 122.
3. Prevent his moving because of risk of fractures. Follow principles on p. 118.
4. See p. 119.
5. Follow principles on p. 119 and let the villain escape.

Chapter 12. Electricity
1. See p. 127. Injury from very high voltage; vehicle in contact with live wire.
2. Possibilities are cessation of breathing and heart beat, brain damage, fractures, burns (pp. 127 and 128).
3. See p. 127.
4. Possible damage to tissues deep to the burn (see p. 128).

Chapter 13. Resuscitation
1. Follow details of steps 1 to 8 on pp. 132 and 133 and of step 11 on p. 128.
2. Prevent anyone trying to 'resuscitate' a patient who is still breathing (pp. 131 and 144).
3. See pp. 144 and 147.
4. See pp. 131 and 144.
5. Quickly clear the sand from the upper part of the body to allow chest movements during resuscitation.
6. Quickly move the patient off the soft bed on to a firm surface before beginning external chest compression (see p. 137).

Chapter 14. Foreign Bodies
1. See p. 152.
2. Advise on wound dressing and on precautions against tetanus (see

p. 151).
3. See p. 152.
4. See p. 151.
5. Refer the boy to hospital or doctor. Put nothing in the ear since its recent infection may have damaged the drum (see p. 152).

Chapter 15. Poisons

1. Suspect poisoning by pesticides (see p. 159).
2. See p. 161. Notify the ambulance service and hospital.
3. Follow steps 4 to 7 of pp. 156 and 157.
4. Follow steps 5 to 7 of pp. 156 and 157. The leader may also decide that this is one of the very rare cases where inducing vomiting is necessary (see p. 157).
5. Study the picture in relation to the text on pp. 162 and 163.

Chapter 16. Animals and Plants

1. Snakebites; other venomous animals (see pp. 167 and 169). Severe reactions to bee stings (see p. 171).
2. He may have been injured by a weever fish or sting ray (see p. 169).
3. See p. 170.

Chapter 17. Heat and Cold

1. P. 184.
2. Hypothermia in a factory where heat has failed overnight. Follow principles on pp. 154 and 155.
3. Pp. 175–6.
4. Pp. 179 and 180.
5. 1 and 3 help to keep warm; 2 and 4 help to keep cool (p. 174).
6. Altered behaviour due to onset of exposure cooling. Adapt treatment principles of p. 182.
7. Heat exhaustion (p. 177). Treat as on p. 178.

Chapter 18. Some Medical Emergencies

1. Behaviour suggests hysteria (see p. 196).
2. See pp. 191 and 192.
3. Suspect low blood sugar in a diabetic on treatment (see p. 197).
4. Epilepsy (see p. 193).
5. Suspect onset of a stroke (see p. 193).
6. Asthma. Ask other passenger to stop smoking. Follow principles on pp. 189 and 190.
7. Suspect heart attack (see p. 191).

Chapter 19. Childbirth

1. See p. 203 and 205.
2. See p. 204 and 207.
3. See p. 207 and 208.
4. See p. 208
5. See p. 209.
6. Suspect possible miscarriage; ask about bleeding (see p. 202).

Chapter 20. Traffic Accidents

1. Motorways and dangerous loads (p. 218).
2. Suspect possible fracture of spine (p. 87). Instruct your friend to support the head. Protect the airway; clear the mouth (p. 110). Remove the helmet (p. 217). Look for possible second (pillion rider) victim (p. 214).
3. See p. 211 to 214. Safeguard against other dangers: p. 215.
4. See p. 214.

Index